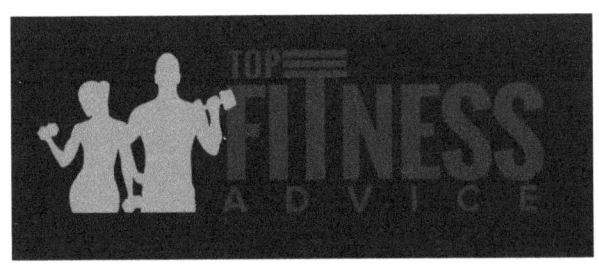

EXERCISE LESS

4th Edition

7-Step Scientifically Proven System to Burn Fat Faster!

LINDA WESTWOOD

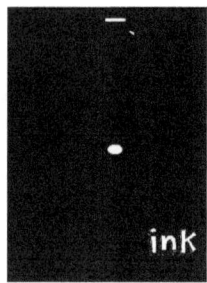

First published in 2015 by Venture Ink Publishing

Copyright © Top Fitness Advice 2019

All rights reserved.

No part of this book may be reproduced in any form without permission in writing from the author. No part of this publication may be reproduced or transmitted in any form or by any means, mechanic, electronic, photocopying, recording, by any storage or retrieval system, or transmitted by email without the permission in writing from the author and publisher.

Requests to the publisher for permission should be addressed to publishing@ventureink.co

For more information about the contents of this book or questions to the author, please contact Linda Westwood at linda@topfitnessadvice.com

Disclaimer

This book provides wellness management information in an informative and educational manner only, with information that is general in nature and that is not specific to you, the reader. The contents of this book are intended to assist you and other readers in your personal wellness efforts. Consult your physician regarding the applicability of any information provided in this book to you.

Nothing in this book should be construed as personal advice or diagnosis, and must not be used in this manner. The information provided about conditions is general in nature. This information does not cover all possible uses, actions, precautions, side-effects, or interactions of medicines, or medical procedures. The information in this book should not be considered as complete and does not cover all diseases, ailments, physical conditions, or their treatment.

You should consult with your physician before beginning any exercise, weight loss, or health care program. This book should not be used in place of a call or visit to a competent health-care professional. You should consult a health care professional before adopting any of the suggestions in this book or before drawing inferences from it.

Any decision regarding treatment and medication for your condition should be made with the advice and consultation of a qualified health care professional. If you have, or suspect you have, a health-care problem, then you should immediately contact a qualified health care professional for treatment.

No Warranties: The author and publisher don't guarantee or warrant the quality, accuracy, completeness, timeliness, appropriateness or suitability of the information in this book, or of any product or services referenced in this book.

The information in this book is provided on an "as is" basis and the author and publisher make no representations or warranties of any kind with respect to this information. This book may contain inaccuracies, typographical errors, or other errors.

Liability Disclaimer: The publisher, author, and other parties involved in the creation, production, provision of information, or delivery of this book specifically disclaim any responsibility, and shall not be held liable for any damages, claims, injuries, losses, liabilities, costs, or obligations including any direct, indirect, special, incidental, or consequences damages (collectively known as "Damages") whatsoever and howsoever caused, arising out of, or in connection with the use or misuse of the site and the information contained within it, whether such Damages arise in contract, tort, negligence, equity, statute law, or by way of other legal theory.

Table of Contents

Disclaimer	3
Who is this book for?	7
What will this book teach you?	9
Introduction	11
Step 1: Choose the Ideal Workout	15
Step 2: Know the HIIT Advantage	23
Step 3: Start Resistance Training to Burn More Calories	31
Step 4: Reap the Rewards of the Ultimate Full Body Workout	47
Step 5: Speed Up Your Progress with Muscle Confusion	81
Step 6: STOP Making these 10 Mistakes Immediately	129
Step 7: Jump Start Your Metabolism with these 10 Tricks	137
Conclusion	149
Final Words	151

Would you prefer to listen to my book, rather than read it?

Download the audiobook version for free!

If you go to the special link below and sign up to Audible as a new customer, you can get the audiobook version of my book completely free.

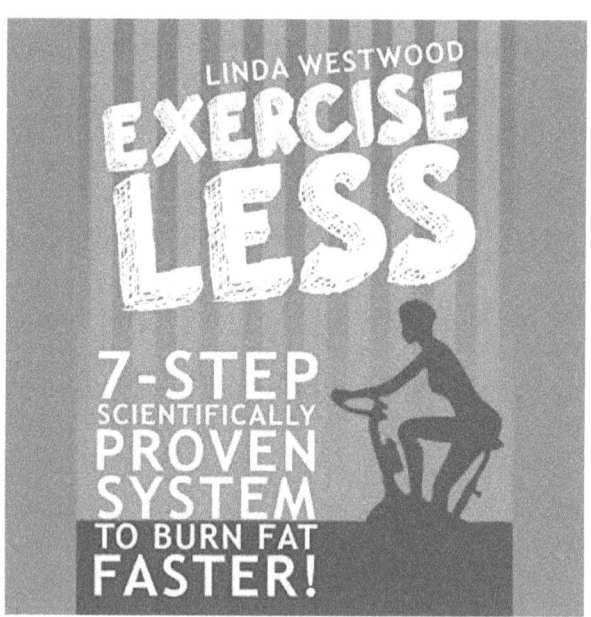

Go here to get your audiobook version for free:

TopFitnessAdvice.com/go/ExerciseLess

Who is this book for?

Do you hate working out because you find it boring?

Are you sick of long, dull workouts that don't bring the results you want?

Do you ever wish you could just workout *less,* but burn *more?*

Then this book is for you!

I am going to share with you some of the MOST effective strategies that you can adopt to start burning up to 300% more calories in your workouts!

You are going to melt fat quicker than ever before!

I have put it all together in a 7-step system that will take you from reading this book to being able to apply the strategies and workouts in your own life!

You can be a complete beginner or someone who works out regularly, it doesn't matter!

If this sounds like you, then keep reading...

What will this book teach you?

This book is not like others!

Inside, I will teach you in great detail how you can start burning up to 300% more calories every day in your workouts!

I go through a fantastic 7-step system that contains everything you need to know, along with the most important tips and strategies.

I also give you several groups of workouts that you can start doing that will burn more calories than your current workout!

Finally, you will learn how you can ALSO burn more calories when you are NOT working out – leading to accelerated fat burning!

Introduction

Whether you are getting older and noticing that your metabolism isn't what it used to be or you have always had trouble keeping the extra pounds off, burning fat and getting in shape is still possible.

You may have tried countless crash diets and more miracle workout routines than you can remember and failed to get the results you want but that doesn't mean that losing weight is a hopeless cause.

If working out has seemed like a long, tedious chore with less than stellar results, you've been doing it all wrong! It's time for a brand-new workout plan that kicks it up a notch—or 300 notches—by shortening the time you spend working out and maximizing the benefits you get from each workout.

The new method is called High Intensity Interval Training (we'll just call it HIIT from here on out). It involves shorter, high intensity workouts instead of long, boring low intensity workouts.

If you're not sure how that could possibly make a difference, keep reading this book to learn the full details.

By following the 7 steps in this book, you can burn as much as 300% more calories every single day. And if that wasn't enough, you'll be working out less than you would have ever thought possible.

This is not some kind of miracle that's too good to be true. It's based on decades of hard science and research. HIIT is not meant to be the lazy person's excuse for a workout. It will take hard work. But that hard work will be compacted into short, highly efficient workouts rather than longer, inefficient (and super boring) workouts that end up just wasting your time when you'd rather be doing anything else.

With HIIT, you can get a full workout done in just 20 minutes and reap the rewards for a full 24 hours afterward. This book will provide you with a step-by-step guide to learn how it works and how you can start making it work for you.

In this book, you'll learn why those longer workouts are waste of your time and totally inefficient. You'll also learn the real science behind why HIIT leads to better results.

In steps 3 through 5, you'll get more information about HIIT as well as 12 complete sample workout plans (6 at the beginner level and 6 at the intermediate level) which you can use exactly as written or modify to better match your needs and skills.

Once you've learned everything you need to know to start your own HIIT workout plan, you'll get even more advice for further maximizing your results.

In step 6, you'll learn how to make your workout even more efficient by avoiding common workout mistakes.

Finally, in chapter 7, you'll learn some extra tricks for boosting your metabolism and burning even more calories.

Don't let yourself get overwhelmed. Take each step one at a time and allow yourself to fully incorporate it before you move on to the next one.

You are much more likely to stick with this new lifestyle for the long term if you make smooth, gradual changes rather than attempt to take it all on at once.

So, work through each step of this book slowly. Give yourself at least one week to make it a complete habit before adding the next step to your routine.

By step 3, you will already start to notice some amazing results!

Burning fat can be fast and fun if you use the HIIT method to boost your metabolism and maximize the number of calories you burn each day.

Get ready to transform your life and feel strong and confident one step at a time!

Step 1

Choose the Ideal Workout

When you think about working out, you are probably imagining long hours at the gym or miles and miles of running through extreme summer heats and frigid winter temperatures.

For centuries, it was believed that the ideal workout was one that was treacherously long and mind-numbingly monotonous. You would have to do the same exact routine over and over, day after day, if you wanted to see results.

Fortunately, scientific studies and innovative workout experts have realized that some traditions are better left in the past. Long, boring, unchanging workouts are one of those traditions that we need to put behind us.

As you'll learn in step 2, shorter, more intense workouts are more effective and have longer lasting effects than long duration, lower intensity workouts.

You'll also learn later how changing up your routine will lead to even faster muscle growth than working out the same muscle groups in the same order day in and day out.

But before we dive into the benefits of high intensity interval trainings and how to use it with cardio, strength training, and what's known as "muscle confusion"; you need to understand why long duration workouts are really a waste of your time.

It's one thing to know that HIIT is an option. But you need to understand why it's the *best* option.

So here are some of the reasons that long duration workouts at a low to moderate intensity are a waste of time, energy, and sanity.

It wastes time

With low intensity workouts, you tend to tack on time rather than step up the intensity. Your workouts get longer and longer as you build endurance.

But by keeping the intensity the same, you're not actually gaining any new strength or muscle mass. You're just maintaining the same level for a longer amount of time.

If you happen to be one of the many people who have other things to do with their lives aside from workout 24/7, there's going to be a point at which you can't afford to keep tacking on time at the end.

More time does not equal more benefits

Even if you do somehow have the time to spend your entire life at the gym, you're not even getting any additional benefit by adding time to your work out.

If you aren't building new muscle mass, you aren't burning any extra calories (beyond what you burn during the workout).

While you may start to see some moderate results after a few weeks on the treadmill, you're quickly going to hit a plateau where you are stuck at the same exact weight, unable to shed those final pounds.

Losing weight doesn't always mean you will lose inches off your waist

If your goal is to fit back into your high school jeans, it's not just a matter of trimming away the extra pounds.

In fact, how much you weigh is one of the least important things. As you might have heard, muscles weigh more than fat but muscle also does a lot more for you than fat.

The more muscle mass you have, the smaller you will be because your muscles are burning your fat for energy. The more muscle you have, the more quickly you burn fat.

So don't shy away from HIIT because you're afraid of bulking up. You need muscle to get thinner. And HIIT doesn't have to bulk you up.

It's boring

You may not immediately think of working out being something fun, but exercise should at least be energizing and exciting. With slow, long duration workouts, you're spending long periods of time doing the same thing. This gets boring fast.

By the end of the first week, the amount of fat you have burned is possibly not going to motivate you enough to endure that kind of mind-numbing boredom for another week.

Even if you do a few different kinds of long duration workouts in a week, they're all going to feel like a dull routine pretty quickly. With such long workout times, you might even start out excited and energized but already become bored halfway through.

You need change, you need bursts of high intensity, and you need shorter workout times to prevent the onset of monotonous boredom.

There's less after burn

After any workout that gets your heart rate elevated, you're also going to get an elevated metabolism. But with low intensity workouts, your metabolism will only stay elevated for a short period of time immediately after the workout.

Once that's over, your metabolism will slow right back down to normal - meaning you'll have to work out again to boost it back up.

No matter how long your low intensity workout lasts, the after burn will be the same – a short period of time immediately after it. This is because you don't have as many muscles to repair (repairing muscles in your body burns extra calories even while you are resting).

While there are many disadvantages, I'm not saying to completely avoid them. If you are an avid runner and enjoy a long run through the park on weekends, do it! If you want to take a nice long dip in the pool and do some slow-paced laps, by all means, go for it!

These low intensity workouts aren't unhealthy or dangerous. They're just not very effective for fat burning or muscle building (which are actually one in the same as you'll soon learn).

So unless the activity is something you enjoy, but instead you're doing it just for the pure sake of doing it and to burn calories, you're wasting your time and your energy.

If you want results, you want to do HIIT.

Go ahead to step 2 to learn more about how and why HIIT workouts are different from low intensity, long duration workouts.

Discover Scientifically-Proven "Shortcuts" & "Hacks" to Lose Weight FASTER (With Very Little Effort)

For this month only, you can get Linda's best-selling & most popular book absolutely free – *Weight Loss Secrets You NEED to Know.*

Get Your FREE Copy Here:
TopFitnessAdvice.com/Bonus

Discover scientifically-proven tips to help you lose weight faster and easier than ever before. With this book, readers were able to improve their weight loss results and fitness levels. So, it's highly recommended that you get this book, especially while it's free!

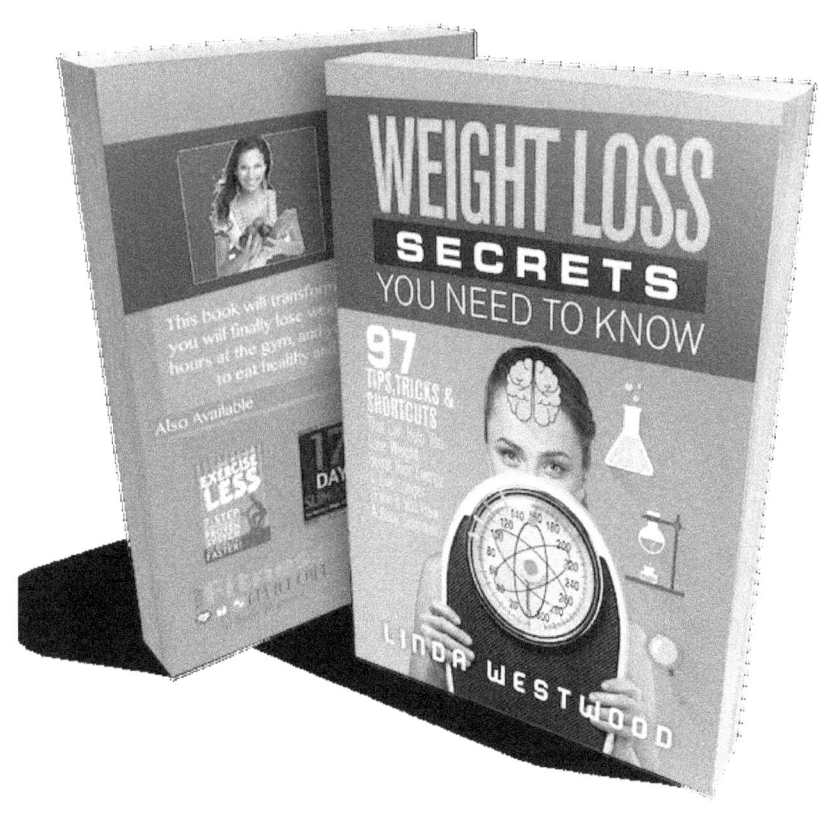

Get Your FREE Copy Here:
TopFitnessAdvice.com/Bonus

Step 2

Know the HIIT Advantage

You might still be thinking long duration, low intensity workouts are more your speed. A lot of people hesitate to try HIIT because the "high intensity" part sounds daunting.

But there are so many benefits to HIIT that you simply cannot get from just doing low intensity cardio (even if you are running a marathon every day).

Just because you might be feeling exhausted and sweaty after a 45-60-minute run doesn't mean you are actually losing weight or burning more calories.

With HIIT, you work out less and get more out of that short period than you do out of your entire long duration cardio routine.

Here are just some of the reasons HIIT is the best option and why everything else is a waste of time (unless you just genuinely enjoy the activity as a hobby, rather than as a workout routine).

Highly Efficient

With a short, 20 minute HIIT workout routine, you can burn more than 200% of the calories you would burn with a 40-minute low intensity workout.

And that's just during the workout itself, you are also going to burn more calories after you're done with an HIIT workout than you would with the longer low intensity workout.

Altogether, you're burning as much as 300% more calories and exercising half the time.

Combine this with our metabolism boosting tricks in step 7, and you could burn well over 300% more calories every single day with a fraction of the time and effort.

Burn More Fat (Even While Resting)

HIIT leads to more total fat burned because it continues to work on your body long after you have stopped working out.

After a 20-minute HIIT workout, your metabolism will remain elevated for a full 24 hours. You'll burn up to 10% more fat just from this extended after burn period than you would with a longer low intensity workout.

The reason this happens is because HIIT focuses on strength; whether it's cardio or weights, you're going to be increasing your strength. This means you are building muscle, or more technically, tearing your muscle tissue so that it needs to be repaired.

Building muscle is a complex process.

After the workout, your muscles will have small tears in them from being pushed to the peak of their ability. Your body will immediately work to repair those tears by building up new muscle fibers (and more muscle fiber than you had before).

To get the extra boost of energy for the additional muscle fiber, your body will be burning *more* energy – hence *more* calories.

What this means for you is: the more muscle you have, the more quickly you will burn fat in the long run, since you're burning energy faster than before.

So if you've been trying long duration cardio workouts and found yourself battling those last stubborn pounds, try HIIT!

Lose Weight without Losing Muscle

Not only is muscle essential for burning fat, you also need it to maintain health and strength.

Many of the low intensity, long duration workout plans end up cutting into your muscle weight more than your actual fat.

This means you might be seeing a lower number on the scale but you still can't seem to get rid of that extra flab around your waistline.

This is especially the case if you combine your low intensity workout with a restrictive diet that focuses on cutting calories rather than boosting nutrition.

With HIIT, you nurture your muscles for a thinner, more toned physique that allows you to lose the weight you actually want to lose (the excess fat that's both unattractive and unhealthy).

HIIT is about maximum efficiency, not hours of suffering at the gym followed by a day of suffering on a restrictive, low calorie diet.

In step 7, you'll get some tips on how to eat (*not* how to diet) so that you are nourishing your body and promoting fat burning while building muscle at the same time. The HIIT workouts you do will leave you feeling strong, confident, and looking better than you have ever looked before.

Boost Your Metabolism

In addition to burning more calories in a shorter amount of time and having a longer after burn period of 24 hours, HIIT will also boost your metabolism.

It does this by increasing the production of HGH (human growth hormone) in your body as much as 450% for the 24 hours after your workout!

Human growth hormone is responsible for telling your metabolism to do its thing (i.e. burn calories). So one short HIIT workout can kick your metabolism into high gear for the rest of the day.

If that's not enough, there's another reason this boost in human growth hormone production is good for you: it slows down the aging process.

That means you'll be looking and feeling younger as your body is better able to repair itself and fight off the decay and degradation of your tissues, bones, and cells.

Maximum Variability

HIIT is not just one kind of exercise. It's a whole workout philosophy. You can apply the same basic principles (burst of high intensity followed by rest or low intensity periods) to absolutely any exercise you like.

Try an HIIT yoga routine (you'll find some options in step 5) or do a powerful 20-minute HIIT weight training routine (found in step 4).

You can even do HIIT with running, swimming, hiking, or anything else that you feel inspired to try. This book alone will give you work out options to do with cardio, weight training, and yoga but don't feel the need to stick with one.

In fact, you'll soon learn why you are better off spicing up your routine by doing a variety of different workouts throughout the week. Mix and match different workouts and you can be sure you never get bored.

Unlimited Potential for Progress

If you do HIIT correctly, you'll be able to make sure you are constantly stimulating muscle growth and burning fat.

With low intensity workouts, your progress will hit a plateau where you are just maintaining the same strength, endurance, and speed week after week. This is because your muscles can predict what's going to happen and because you aren't pushing them to work harder (at most, you're just pushing them to work longer).

With HIIT, you'll start making progress quickly and you'll be able to continue making progress.

Get Stronger Bones and Joints

The emphasis on strength with HIIT has been proven to not only build muscle but also increase bone density. This will make your bones less brittle and breakable and as you get older, the higher bone density will help prevent osteoporosis.

In addition to muscle and bone density, HIIT workouts also build strong connective tissues, which provide sturdy support to your joints. This could lower your risk for arthritis and a host of other joint problems.

Build a Lean Body

If you do an exclusively low intensity cardio workout, you're going to hit a point where you plateau as mentioned earlier.

You won't get any new muscle and you might actually risk losing muscle (especially if you're also eating a low protein diet in an effort to cut those final pounds).

Depriving yourself of nutrition and muscle-building exercises is going to lead you to become "skinny fat". That is, you'll look thin but you won't be toned (and you'll be at high risk for many health problems that you might think only affect obese people).

With HIIT, you combine high intensity cardio, strength training, and muscle confusion to make sure that you are building and strengthening your muscles.

Muscle will burn more fat in the long run (as I previous said) and will make you not only stronger but also leaner and thinner. You'll have a toned, lean body without any flabby or loose skin that comes from just losing fat without gaining muscle. Remember, though, muscle weighs more than fat so don't measure your progress in pounds, measure it in inches. Give yourself a goal waistline rather than a goal weight.

All of these benefits are achievable with a good HIIT workout plan. But it is important to note that because HIIT does involve high intensity exercise (even though it's for short bursts), you need to approach with caution.

If you do not currently have any kind of workout plan, you need to start from the beginning and work your way up. Gradually build up to a full HIIT program so that you can avoid serious injury or permanent damage.

You wouldn't suddenly go to the gym and try to lift a 250-pound weight if you've never done weightlifting a day in your life. So don't dive head first into an advanced HIIT workout if you haven't already been working out for a while.

Even if you start at the beginner level, you're still going to see fast and impressive results. If you stick with it and progress at a pace that feels right for you, you'll see that you are exercising like a pro within a couple months.

You should also remember to give yourself rest days. A good cycle for the week is to do 2 days on and 1 day off. That is, 2 days of HIIT workouts and 1 day of rest. If you are feeling extra motivated, your rest day can be a day of low intensity exercise (go for an even paced jog or do a few laps in the pool at a moderate speed).

If you do go for this second option, just make sure that your low intensity day is not one where you push yourself to your maximum limit.

Just get your heart pumping and leave it at that. Your muscles need time to repair and build so you don't want to constantly push them to the point of strain every single day.

Now that you have learned about the benefits of HIIT and why it's the best option, no matter who you are, it's time to move on to step 3.

Step 3 will focus on applying the HIIT workout structure to cardio exercises. You'll get your first set of sample workout routines (for the beginner and intermediate levels) and you'll see how to put the amazing powers of HIIT into practice.

I hope that you are enjoying this book so far, and if you could spare 30 seconds, I would greatly appreciate you leaving a review on Amazon.com.

Step 3

Start Resistance Training to Burn More Calories

Earlier in this book, you may have gotten the impression that cardio is a waste of time and that HIIT is all about hitting the weights hard.

This is absolutely not true.

HIIT can be used with any kind of exercise whether it's cardio based or weight based. The HIIT advantage has more to do with *how* you do that exercise, not what the exercise is.

In step 3, you'll see how adding resistance to your cardio routine will maximize your results and shorten the time you spend on the treadmill, elliptical, or stationary bike.

First, we'll take a look at what it means to add resistance and what the benefits of doing so are.

Then, you'll get 4 separate and complete workout routines that you can either replicate entirely or modify to better suite your needs.

Why Resistance is the Key to Cardio

Resistance is what adds strength training to your cardio routine. By adding strength training, you are turning your bland cardio workout into an all-in-one cardiovascular and muscle building exercise that will get every system in your body working at full capacity.

You are combining all the benefits of weight lifting with all the benefits of cardio into one single workout.

Resistance cardio essentially takes your normal cardio activity and makes it more challenging by adding resistance in some way. For example, running on a flat surface is just plain cardio. But running uphill on an incline is resistance cardio.

This is because you are not only propelling yourself forward; you are working to lift your bodyweight upward to get up the hill at the same time.

On a bicycle, you add resistance by changing the gears so that you have to peddle harder to go the same distance. This resistance means that you are using more muscle than you normally would to do the same exact activity.

That's where the strength training comes in.

Some of the benefits of doing resistance cardio include:

- Burning fat faster
- Better mood
- Stronger immune system
- Increased stamina
- Healthier muscles
- Stronger heart
- Better circulation
- Stronger lungs

- Decrease in body pain
- Stronger bones
- Stronger joints
- Younger appearance
- More energy throughout the day

Each of the following workouts are using running as the cardio activity. But if you don't like running, you can also use the same basic framework of each of these workouts with another cardio activity.

Here are some examples of other cardio activities that will work and might be more exciting for you than running:

- Swimming
- Cycling
- Jumping jacks
- Rollerblading
- Dancing
- Zumba
- Hiking
- Snowshoeing
- Rowing machine
- Cross country skiing
- Surfing
- Most sports
- Jumping on a trampoline

And that's just a few of your options. There are literally hundreds of cardio exercises that you can do with HIIT. Just find one you like and remember to alternate between high intensity and low intensity intervals at the right times.

Beginner Resistance Workouts

The beginner works out are starting you out at a 1:2 ratio. That means your rest or low intensity interval will be twice as long as your high intensity interval during your workout.

Typically: 20 seconds of high intensity for 40 seconds of low intensity or rest. If you find that 20 seconds of high intensity is still too much for you right now, lower it to 10 or 15 seconds and add the time you cut from that to your low intensity interval.

If you find that it's not enough and you want to push yourself a little harder, you can bump it up to 25 seconds or even skip right on up to the intermediate level (1:1 or 30 seconds of high intensity with 30 seconds of low intensity).

The important thing is that you push yourself but never push yourself to the breaking point.

The first moment that you feel like you want to stop, push yourself for 3 to 5 seconds past that. If you continue to just push yourself a little further in this way, you'll progress quickly without risking a serious injury.

Outside the Gym

Getting your workout done outside the gym means you get to enjoy fresh air and sunlight, but it means you can't regulate your pace or time your intervals as easily. Use a stopwatch (or the stopwatch function on your smartphone) to time your intervals.

On some watches, you can set it to make a sound at different intervals, which will save you from having to reset it during your workout. If that's not possible, just reset it yourself during your rest interval or have a friend time you.

Now, onto the outdoor workout

Go to a public basketball court or a park with a court-sized asphalt area that you can use. Bring a basketball.

Start with a short warm up.

Do 10 laps of a brisk walk or light jog around the court while dribbling the basketball slowly (just fast enough that you can keep it with you as you walk or jog).

Alternate your dribbling hand with each lap.

It may take a while to get used to dribbling with your non-dominant hand but you'll get the hang of it.

An added benefit is that it has been proven through research that use of our non-dominant hand for various tasks, such as this one, increases brain function and development.

Along the outer border of the court, do squat shuffles (you'll read about these in step 4). Instead of going from side to side and touching the ground, do a full lap of squat shuffles around the court while dribbling a basketball as quickly as you can without losing control.

Dribble it from one hand to the other so that they are both working throughout the exercise. Once you have completed one full lap around, squat shuffle to the other side so that your legs get a balanced workout.

Do high intensity intervals for 20 seconds and low intensity intervals for 40 seconds.

High intensity in this case means squatting as low as you can without falling over and shuffling to the side as quickly as you can.

Low intensity can be just walking if you are completely exhausted. If you want more of a challenge, just lift out of the squat a little more and shuffle a little slower.

Repeat this cycle of intervals for a total of 20 times. Then do a cool down walk or light jog while dribbling slowly for 10 laps (exactly as you did in the warm up). Altogether it will be between 25 and 30 minutes.

By adding the basketball here, you are doing a full body cardio workout. The squat position will build strength and provide the resistance you need even though you are on a flat surface.

Dribbling the ball will build coordination and work as light resistance cardio for your arms.

If timing the intervals during this workout does not seem possible, you can use the basketball court as a rough gauge. Do high intensity along one long edge and then low intensity around the other three sides. As you get better, you can do high intensity for one long edge and one short edge and low intensity for the other two edges.

If you use this method instead of time, just make sure you keep count and get 20 high intensity intervals in and 20 low intensity intervals (that will be 20 total laps around the full court).

At the Gym

In this exercise, you'll use the treadmill.

Start with a 5-minute warm up walk. It should be a brisk pace but you shouldn't be running just yet (somewhere between 3-5mph).

Raise the incline of your treadmill somewhere between 5% and 10% - whatever you can handle running on at a high speed for 20 seconds.

Then bump up the speed to the fastest that you can handle without flying off the treadmill. Run at this speed for 20 seconds.

Lower the incline to 0%. Slow down to a brisk walk or light jog (4-6mph) for 40 seconds.

Repeat this 20 second/40 second cycle of high intensity and low intensity 20 times total.

Cool down with a brisk 5-minute walk. It should be at the same pace as your warm up walk.

Step off the treadmill and do some stretches. Focus on stretching your hamstrings and other leg muscles.

Altogether, this will take you about 30 minutes: 5 minutes of warm up, 20 minutes of workout, 5 minutes of cool down, and finally a couple of minutes for stretching.

This workout primarily targets the muscles in the lower body. It will result in fat loss throughout your whole body, though, because the body uses the fat stores from everywhere as fuel.

But if you want to do a full body workout, you can add a quick 10-minute upper body cardio workout. Do this before you do your 5-minute cool down.

Do a quick 1-2-minute stretch focusing on your arms, shoulders and upper back.

Find a punching bag and wrap your hands or wear gloves.

Get into a firm boxing stance - legs slightly wider than hip width apart with one leg slightly in front of you and one leg slightly back, knees slightly bent, elbows bent so that your fists are just above your heart.

When in the correct stance, start boxing – punching the bag like it's everyone who ever made your life difficult all wrapped into one evil, annoying bag!

Continue to punch with everything you've got for 20 seconds. Then rest or punch air for 40 seconds. Repeat this cycle 10 times.

If there isn't a punching bag at your gym, you can hold light weights (no more than 3 to 5 pounds) and just punch air while holding them, alternating between 20 seconds of high intensity, rapid punching and 40 seconds of low intensity slower punches (you can drop the weights during the low intensity punches).

Remember to do a cool down walk after this while stretching your arms.

This will bring your total time at the gym up to about 40 minutes.

If you'd prefer to keep your daily gym time down, you can alternate days of upper and lower body cardio. But remember to always have one rest or low intensity day for every two HIIT days.

Intermediate Resistance Workouts

For an intermediate level resistance workout, you can choose to do either of the beginner workouts if they appeal to you more than the 2 you are about to read below.

Just up the challenge by doing 30 seconds of high intensity and 30 seconds of low intensity or rest (repeat that 20 times).

Otherwise, try one of the following specially designed intermediate workouts.

Outside the Gym

For the intermediate outdoor resistance workout, we're going to try something that's both challenging and fun. You can make the world your playground by using outdoor objects in new ways to get an awesome workout that never gets boring.

To start, estimate a 2 ½ mile route through your neighborhood, town, large park or some sort of area that you can run through.

Alternatively, do a 1 ¼ mile route that you will go in both directions.

Get out a pen and paper.

Pick 4 or 5 landmarks or objects that you know will be on your path: fire hydrants, benches, bicycle, a certain kind of tree, whatever you like.

They should be things you know you'll see but that won't be so common you'll see them every step of the way.

For example, don't choose "tree" if you plan on running in a forest.

For each landmark or object you list, assign it a specific exercise: pushups, shoulder presses, or pretty much any of the other exercises from step 3 that doesn't require equipment.

Now, get out and start running.

Remember to warm up first by briskly walking or lightly jogging the first ¼ mile of your route. Then, break into your fastest sprint for 20 seconds.

If you don't have a timer, just count out 20 seconds in your head. Remember to count slowly by saying something like "1-1,000-2-1,000" and so on. Don't let your counting speed up because you're trying to rush to stop.

After your 20 seconds of high intensity running is up, give yourself a 40 second low intensity break (just walk or jog at a moderate pace).

Each time you see one of your landmarks or objects, stop and do a set of 10 repetitions of whichever exercise was assigned to that object.

Repeat this for the next 2 miles of your route.

Do a cool down walk or light jog for the last ¼ mile. Altogether, you'll be doing a ¼ mile warm up, a 2-mile workout (with random breaks for exercises based on your landmarks), and a ¼ mile cool down for a total of 2 ½ miles.

This workout is naturally a resistance workout since running outdoors means you'll be dealing with uneven terrain. But you can increase the resistance by purposely picking a route that includes a lot of hills so that you can do more incline running.

The benefits of this workout structure are not only that it stays exciting by virtue of the fact that you're not entirely sure when to expect one of your marked objects to pop up; but it also works as muscle confusion (which you will learn more about in step 5).

By stopping at completely random points to do a different kind of exercise that works out a different group of muscles, your entire body will stay on alert and get a full workout.

Keep things fresh and exciting by changing your list of landmarks or objects, changing which exercises are associated with them, or going on a different route.

When you start to notice that getting through the full 2 ½ mile route is getting too easy, you can add on more distance.

At the Gym

Working out at the gym might not be as exciting as the intermediate outdoor resistance workout that you just read about above but it will be easier to time your intervals and track your progress.

For this workout, you'll use an elliptical machine or similar stair stepping machine and a resistance band. The resistance band is essentially just a long elastic band. So get a resistance band and get onto an elliptical machine.

Start at a moderate pace for 5 minutes to warm up.

Then, wrap your resistance band around the console or body of the elliptical and hold one end in each hand. Now, set the machine to either the highest incline or the highest resistance.

Different models will allow for either increased resistance or increased incline. Some models may allow you to adjust both, in that case, just pick one or the other to max out.

Once it's at the highest level, pump as hard as you can with your legs for 30 seconds. While you are moving your legs, pull the resistance band toward yourself. Pull with one arm at a time as far back as you can. After the 30 seconds is up, decrease the resistance or incline back down and do your 30-second low intensity interval.

Repeat the high intensity and low intensity interval cycle 20 times (for a total of 20 minutes). Then do a 5-minute cool down at the same pace as your warm up.

After your cool down, take a few minutes to stretch. You'll want to do stretches for your arms, legs, and back.

Altogether, this should take about 30 minutes.

By combining your time on the elliptical with the resistance band, you're getting a full body resistance cardio workout so you'll get everything covered in that 30 minutes.

There are some models of elliptical machines that come with resistance bands already attached but even if the one you are using doesn't, you can still use a separate resistance band. This workout can also be easily adapted to a stationary bike.

In this chapter, you've already gotten four great resistance cardio workouts, which combine cardio with some resistance training. But, resistance cardio can't be a complete substitute for a solid strength-training workout.

So in the next chapter, you'll learn about strength training with and without equipment so that you can target muscle growth to increase the amount of fat you can burn in a day.

Remember, the best workout plans combine different kinds of exercises to create a balanced routine that takes care of the whole body and helps prevent predictability.

So don't just pick one workout from this entire book. Combine at least one workout from each step and modify them as necessary to create the ideal balance of strength, cardio, and flexibility for the ultimate fat burning workout plan.

Once again, thank you for reading this book, and I hope you're getting a lot of valuable information. I would greatly appreciate it if you could take 30 seconds to leave me a review for this book on Amazon.com.

Enjoying this book?

Check out my other best sellers!

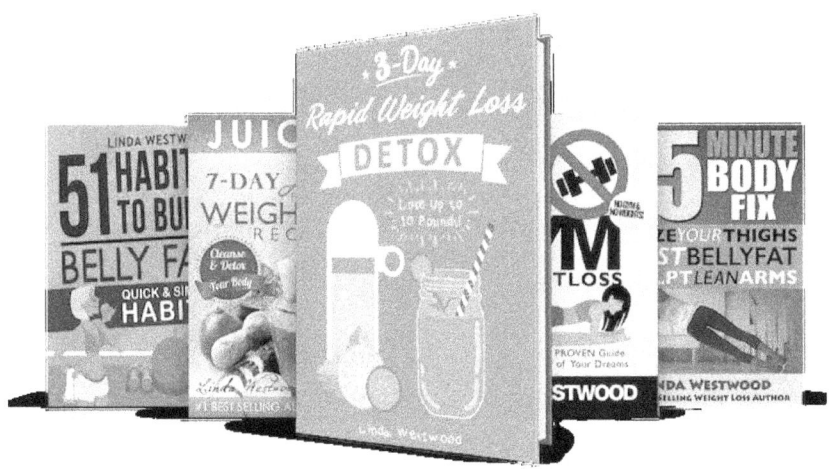

Get your next book on sale here:

TopFitnessAdvice.com/go/books

Step 4

Reap the Rewards of the Ultimate Full Body Workout

So far, you have learned how HIIT is more effective than long duration (lower intensity) workouts.

More importantly, you have learned *why* HIIT is more effective and how it works on your body to maximize calories burned and muscles worked. You've also read through some suggested workout routines with both beginner and intermediate exercises.

These workout routines have been mainly focused on cardio activities with increasing levels of resistance to help burn more calories and burn more fat.

But it's equally important to include a good strength-training workout into your weekly routine (at least 1-2 days per week).

In this chapter, you are going to learn about weight training and strength training.

But the difference here is that you will be doing full body strength training workouts rather than just focusing on one part of the body or one group of muscles.

In this way, your strength training sessions will have a bit of cardio blended in, which will boost the number of calories burned and keep your metabolic rate elevated long after the workout.

First, let's talk about why strength training is essential for weight loss.

Most people think of strength training or weight training just as a way of bulking up. And those who don't want to bulk up tend to stay far away from the weights or any exercise that they think will give them monstrous biceps or quads. But the fact is, muscle helps you burn fat.

The more muscle you have, the higher your resting metabolic rate will be which means you will burn more calories on average throughout the day even if you were to spend an entire day in bed.

Building muscle in addition to burning fat is what will allow you to break out of a plateau and continue moving toward your ideal weight.

If you only focus on fat loss, you are going to get very frustrated when you notice that you are not getting the same amazing results from your workouts that you saw at the beginning.

With that in mind, you might be thinking, "sure, that sounds fine but I don't want to go start lifting weights at the gym next to those big bulky guys!"

Well, the good news is you don't have to.

In this chapter (just as with the other chapters), you'll get your non-gym alternative for each experience level.

It is possible to do full body strength training workouts without a single piece of equipment. You can also do the gym version at home if you're willing to shell out the cash for some quality home gym equipment.

Remember - test your personal abilities with each exercise before committing to any routine. You can do this by doing sets of 10 for each exercise in the workout.

However, many full sets of 10 you can do right now is the number of sets you should start with. Gradually increase the number of sets, as you get stronger.

Always remember to include a 5-minute warm up before your work out and a 5-minute cool down after you finish.

The warm up should be more cardio focused because the purpose of a warm up is to get your blood pumping through your muscles and get fluid into your joints so that they are protected from damage.

You can do jumping jacks, jump rope, or a quick, low intensity jog on the treadmill.

Whatever you choose, it shouldn't be high intensity and it shouldn't involve heavy weights. You are just trying to get warmed up, not worn out.

Your 5-minute cool down after the workout should just involve stretching.

Wiggle out your arms and legs to loosen the muscles and do some stretches while everything is still warm. This will help you avoid muscle cramps and tears by keeping your muscles stretched and flexible.

Beginner Full Body Workouts

Remember to rest between each set for the same amount of time you spent on the set. If it took you 30 seconds, rest 30 seconds. If it took you 60 seconds, rest 60 seconds.

In the beginning stages, high intensity intervals should be the same length of time as your rest intervals. As you progress, you can decrease the rest intervals.

A good rate of decrease is to cut 10 seconds off your rest intervals each week. But always work at a pace that suits your needs.

If you need to spend 2 weeks at the same pace, do it. This will benefit you more in the long run than pushing yourself too hard.

If you push too hard, you could end up injuring yourself, which could knock you out of the game for weeks and completely kill your momentum.

At Home

1. Tuck Jumps (3x10)

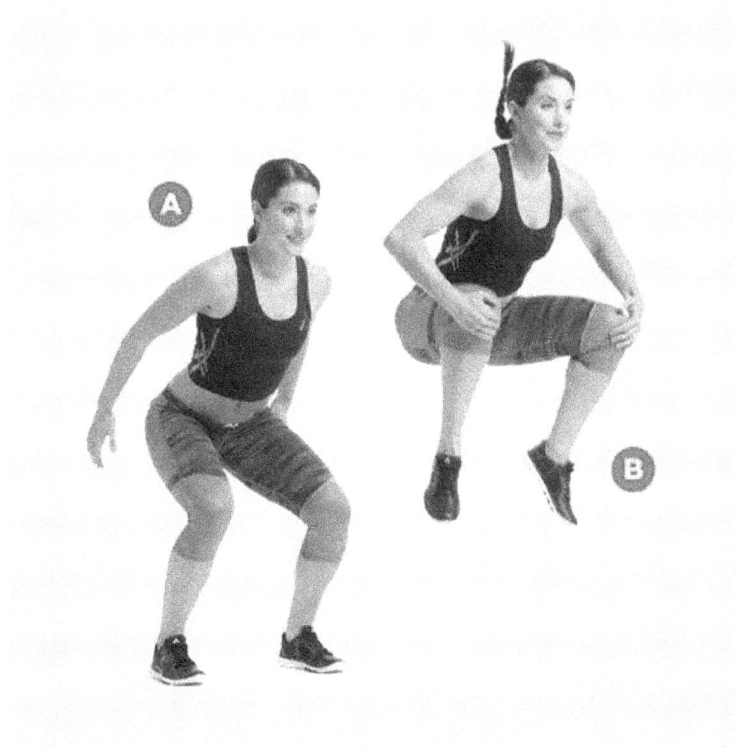

Tuck jumps combine muscle toning and cardio into one fun and quick exercise. To do it, stand straight with knees slightly bent.

Jump as high as you can while pulling the knees in toward your chest. Land with knees slightly bent and jump again.

During this entire time, keep your arms straight out in front of you, parallel to the ground. For added intensity, hold two small weights in your hands.

2. Plank (3x60 seconds)

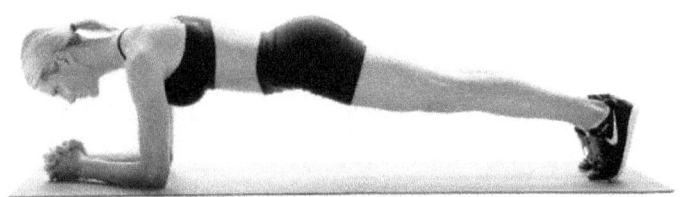

This move is one of the primary positions in yoga. To do it, get down into a push up position. Let your elbows bend down until your forearms are flat against the floor.

Interlace your fingers. Your knees and spine should be straight. Don't let your butt lift up. Your body should be one flat plank. Keep your neck straight as well.

Don't let it hang down. Hold this position for 60 seconds.

If you can do it for longer, do it. Despite the fact that you don't have to do any repetitions for this, it's still a surprisingly dynamic post that keeps your abs, thighs, arms, chest, neck and back all fully engaged the entire time.

3. Lunge with Arms Raised (2x20)

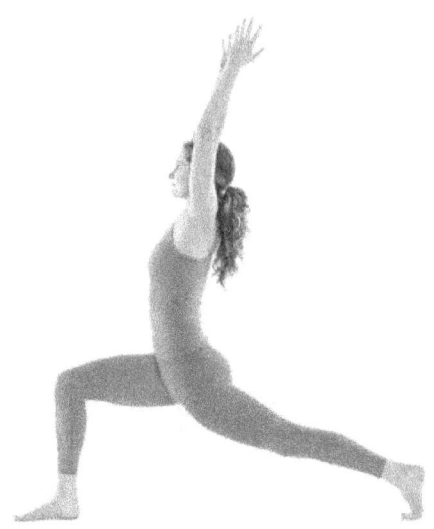

This is a fairly well known strength-training move. And it became so well-known because it is extremely effective - especially for the thighs and calves.

To do it, start by standing up straight. Raise your arms straight out in front of you.

Step one leg forward about 2 or 3 feet in front of you (as far as you can go without falling over) and bend your knee into it until your thigh is about parallel with the ground.

Keep the back leg straight and push the heel toward the ground. Hold the lunge for about 10 seconds.

Step your back leg forward to stand up straight again. Do the same with the other leg. Alternate between legs likes this throughout each set so that each one gets an even workout. Keep your arms raised the entire time.

4. *Dolphin Push Up (2x10)*

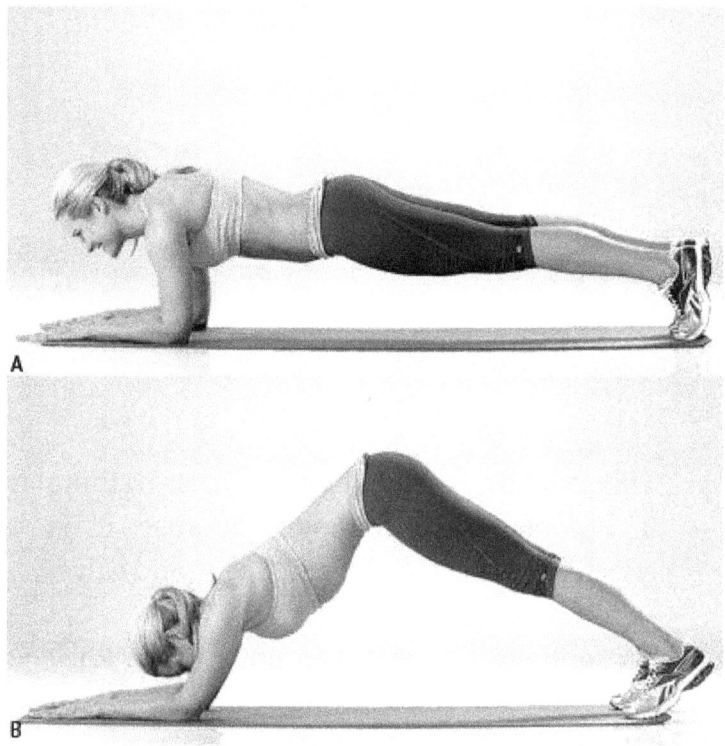

This one is great for your arms, shoulders, upper back and abs but it also does wonders for your legs. Start in downward dog position (the most popular yoga position).

Press your elbows downward until your forearms are resting on the floor. While your arms are in this position, lift your heels up and come onto your toes.

Push your heels back down toward the floor. Push your elbows up and return to the original down dog position. Each full cycle through this is one repetition.

Repeat 10 times and then take a short 15-20 second rest in downward dog position before doing another set of 10.

5. *Superman (3x30 seconds)*

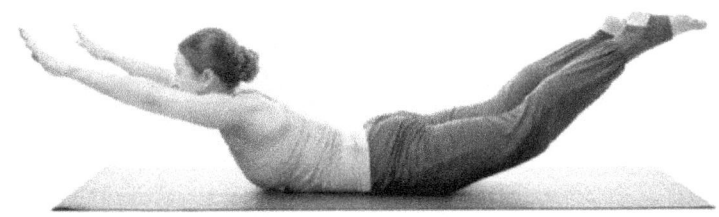

This position looks deceivingly simple but it is actually extremely dynamic and keeps your full body working. To do it, lie down on your stomach.

Raise your arms above your head with your palms on the floor. In one breath, raise your arms and legs off the floor as high as you can so that you are balancing on your belly.

Hold this position for 30 seconds or longer if you can. You can kick this one up a notch by adding ankle weights and holding weights in your arms.

6. Boxer (5x10)

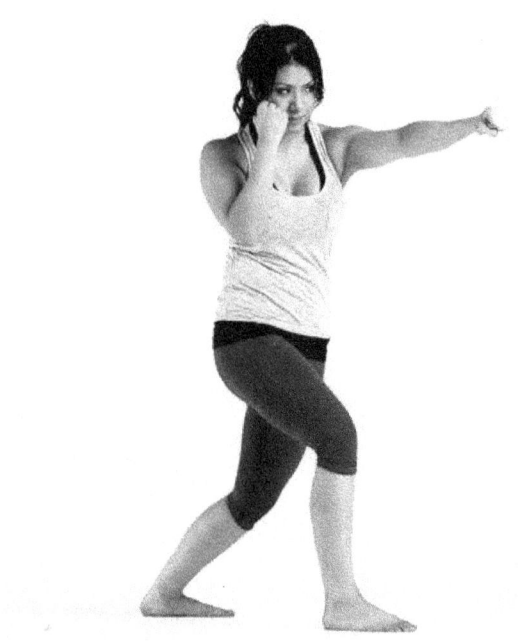

This active pose gives you a full body workout without requiring too much balance. It's pretty simple to perform but will give you a surprisingly effective workout.

Start by standing with your legs hip width apart and your knees bent about 45 degrees (when you get better, you can do a full 90-degree chair squat).

Bend forward from your waist so that your torso is parallel to the ground.

Keep your spine straight and look at the ground. Punch one arm straight in front of you as you punch the other arm straight behind you. Hold the arms in that position for one breath and then alternate arms.

At the Gym

This one can be done at the gym, or at home if you have a pair of dumbbells. It is recommended to do it at the gym, though, because then you can gradually increase the weight as you progress to keep it challenging.

1. *The Skier (60 seconds)*

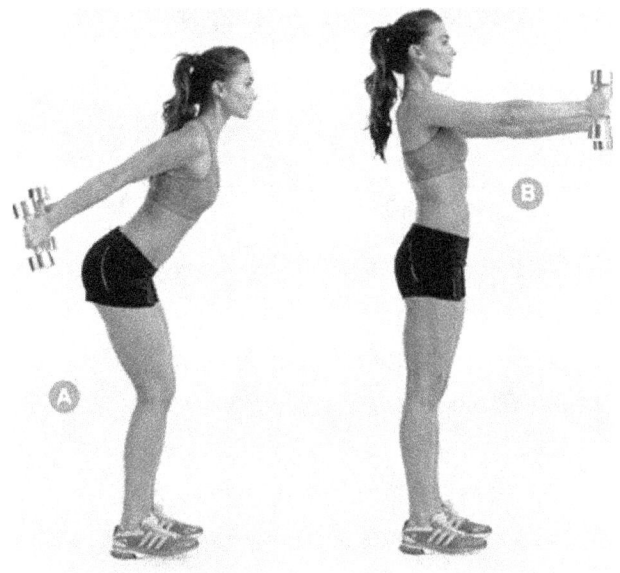

Hold a 3 to 5-pound weight in each hand. Stand straight with your arms to your side. Lift your arms straight out in front of you.

Then slowly swing your arms behind you while bending over so that your torso is parallel to the ground. You'll look like a stationary skier (hence the name).

Make sure your knees are slightly bent so that they don't lock.

2. *Plank to Push Up (60 seconds)*

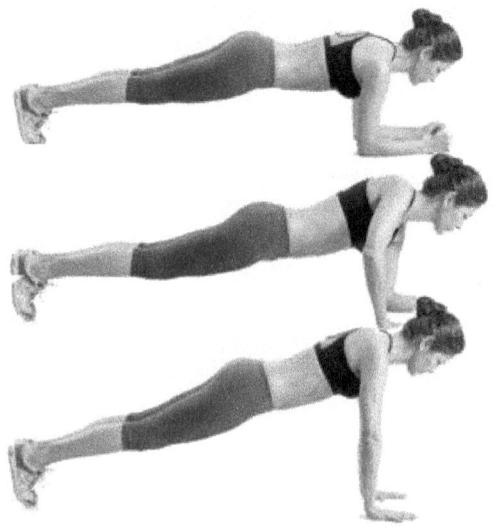

This move is described in the intermediate at home workout below.

If you need to modify it, use a step platform or similar object to place your hands on so that you don't have to sink as low into the plank.

3. *Squat Thrust with Dumbbells (60 seconds)*

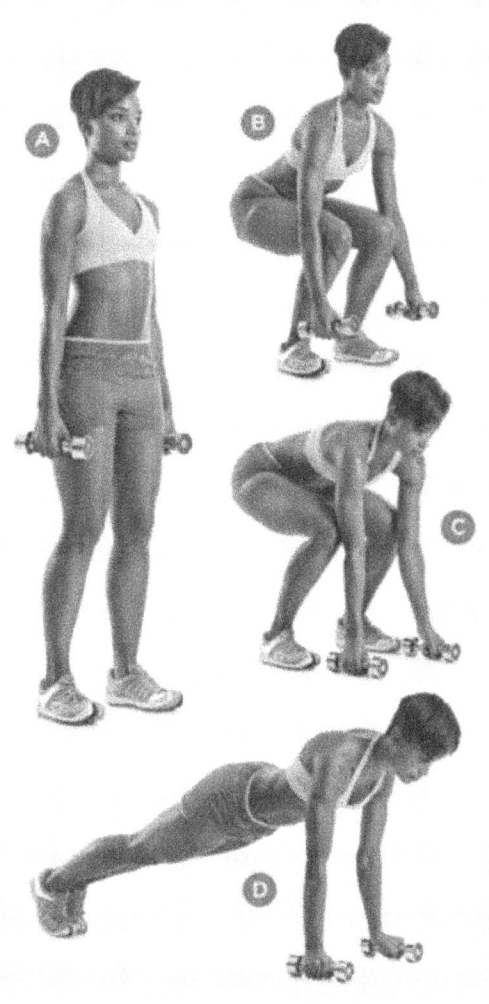

For this exercise, you will stand with your legs hip width apart. Hold a 3 to 5-pound weight in either hand. Squat down and press the weights into the floor.

Your arms should be straight with elbows slightly bent. Place your bodyweight onto your arms as you jump your legs backward into a push up position.

Then jump your legs back up to a squatting position and then stand up straight again. Move through this sequence in one fluid but controlled motion.

If you want to make it more challenging, you can do a push up when your legs are back in push up position.

4. *Shoulder Press with Squats (60 seconds)*

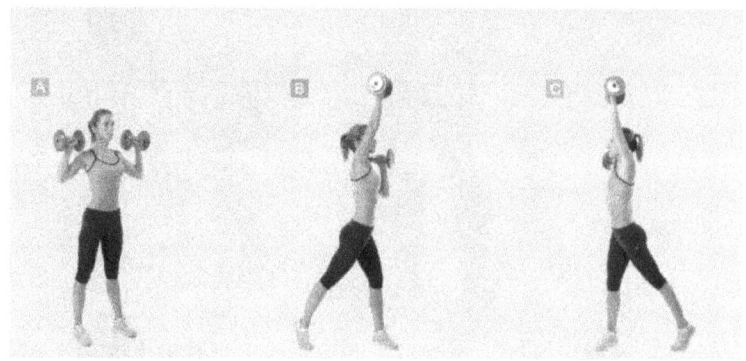

For this one, you are going to start with your weights in your hands and your elbows bent so that your weights are level with your ears (like you are ready to box someone).

As you push one weight straight above you, twist your hips toward the side opposite the arm you are lifting.

As you pull your weight back down to hip level, straighten your hips and push down into a squat.

Come back up from the squat and do the same thing in the other direction with your other arm.

Continue to alternate arms (remembering to squat between rotations) for the full 60 seconds.

5. *Squat Shuffle (60 seconds)*

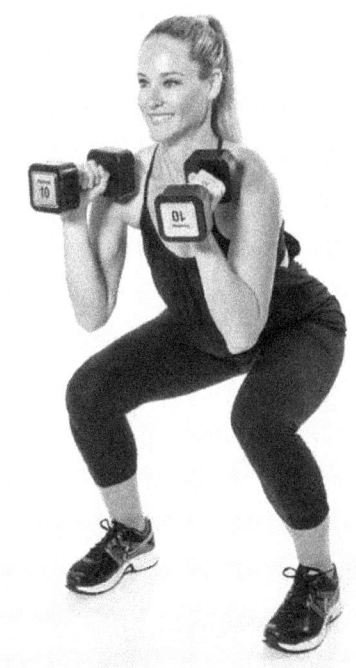

Start with your legs wider than hip width apart. Squat down. Bend your elbows up and hold your weights in front of your chest.

While keeping your legs constantly in squat position, move your left leg out to the side and bring your right leg in so that you are shuffling to the left side.

Take 3 shuffle steps like this and then touch the floor with the weight in your left hand.

Take 3 shuffle steps to the right and then touch the floor with the weight in your right hand.

Repeat this series of 5 moves 3 to 5 times. Don't take any breaks between exercises but do give yourself a 5-minute break after going through all 5 moves.

Each round is designed to last 5 minutes (60 seconds per exercise). Because it's based on time rather than a set number of repetitions, you should do as many as you can do within the 60 seconds given for each exercise.

Don't speed through it though.

The most important thing is to pay attention to form and make sure you are completing the full exercise correctly.

Fewer repetitions done correctly will be more effective in the long run than a lot of incorrectly done repetitions. Plus, there's less danger of hurting yourself.

Intermediate Full Body Workouts

You are ready to step up your game and move to intermediate level workouts when you can handle high intensity intervals that are longer than your rest intervals. You want to lengthen the high intensity interval as you shorten the rest interval.

Typically, you can say you are ready for an intermediate level workout if you can do 45 seconds of high intensity with 25-30 second rest intervals.

After more training, you'll reach the goal ratio of 2:1. That is, your rest intervals will be half as long as your high intensity intervals.

This usually looks like 60 seconds of high intensity for 30 seconds of rest. At the most advanced stage, your rest interval will not be just sitting or standing around; it'll be low intensity exercise.

In a strength-training routine, cut the weight by half and do the same moves you were doing at high intensity but for half the time. Then go back to full weight and do it for the full time.

At Home

1. *Headstand Push Up (1x10)*

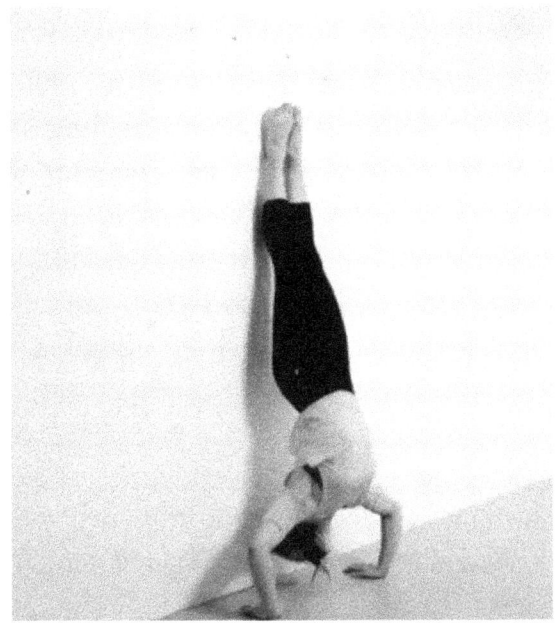

This one will impress all your friends while also maximizing the benefits you would get from a regular push up. This one puts more weight on your arms (for even more muscle strengthening) while also giving your whole body a workout.

You'll need to keep your abs, back, legs and chest muscles taught to keep yourself balanced in this pose. So, to start, you'll need to get in headstand position against a wall.

To do this, start in a dolphin push up position (forearms flat against the floor, butt in the air) with your head about 8-10 inches from the wall. Slowly walk your feet up toward your head.

Then when you can't walk them any closer, gently push off until you feel your butt hit the wall.

With your butt leaning against the wall, raise your feet straight up until your feet are resting against the wall. Let your head rest gently between your arms.

Carefully push one arm up at a time while allowing most of your body weight to rest against the wall. Once both of your arms are straightened and your head is lifted off the floor, you are ready to start doing pushups.

Lower your arms to a 90-degree angle, hold for one breath and then straighten them again (holding for one breath when they are straight).

Be careful not to lock your elbows at any point. And do not try to do this pose quickly.

Do it slowly so that you are focusing as much on balance as you are on completing the push up.

2. *Arm Circles (2x45seconds)*

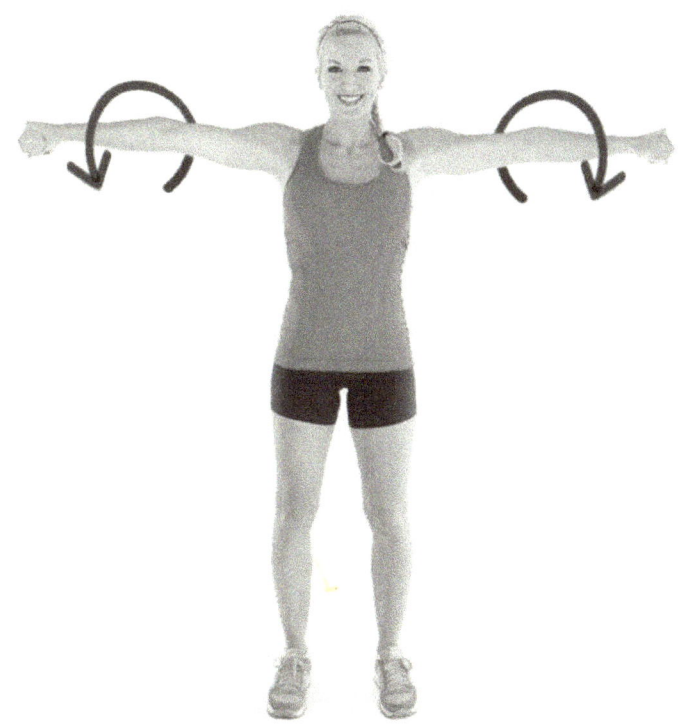

This one looks so simple it will seem like you are hardly doing anything at all but once you do your first 45 second rep, you'll realize how misleading appearances can be.

While in full lunge, stick your arms straight out to the sides so that you are making a T shape. Rotate them clockwise for 45 seconds.

Stand up straight; take a 15-20-minute breather and then lunge with the other leg.

This time, rotate your arms counter clockwise for 45 seconds. To give yourself an added challenge, do this while holding weights in your hands.

3. *Plyometric Push Up (3x10)*

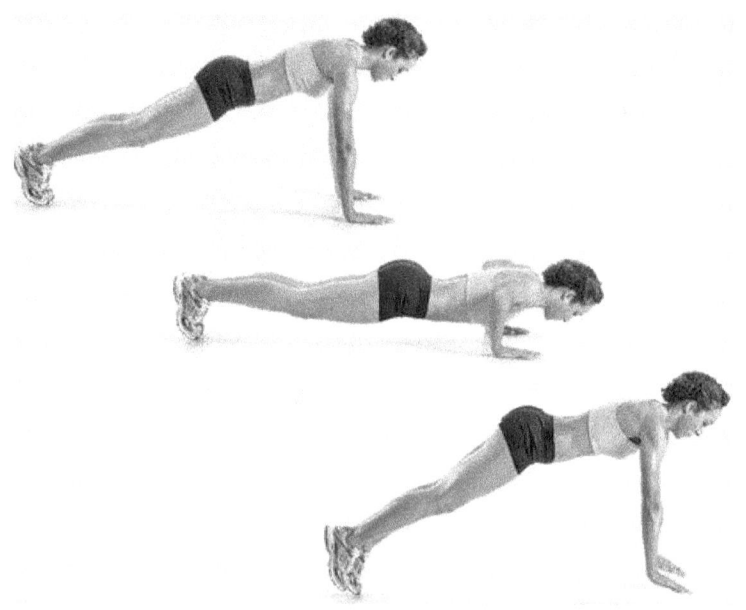

This is the traditional push up on steroids. Get into position as if you were doing a normal push up.

Bend your arms to come down. When you go back to the up position, do it with an explosion of force so that your hands push off the ground entirely and you are suspended in the air for a split second.

Once your hands hit the ground again, immediately bend your elbows and go down into the next push up.

This will give you the strength training of a traditional push up with a little more cardio to it so that you can kick start your metabolism at the same time.

4. *Triceps Dip with Leg Raise (4x10)*

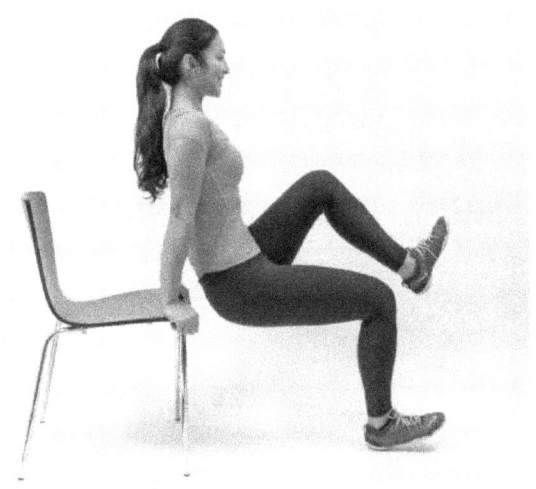

This one is particularly great for your arms, back, shoulders, and chest. The added leg raises will give benefits to your legs and abs while also adding a cardio element to the exercise.

Start by sitting on the edge of your bed or a sturdy chair/coffee table. You'll be pushing down on the edge with a good amount of force so make sure it's not something that's going to flip over.

Stick your legs out straight so that just the heels are on the floor. Straighten your elbows and push your palms down as you raise yourself off the bed or chair.

Raise one leg up as high as you can while keeping it completely straight. Hold it up like this as you push down until your but nearly reaches the floor (or until your elbows form a 90-degree angle).

Push your arms back up straight. Keep the same leg raised for the full set of 10. Switch to the other leg for the next set of 10. Alternate until you have done 2 sets of 10 for each leg.

5. *Plank to Push Up (3x10)*

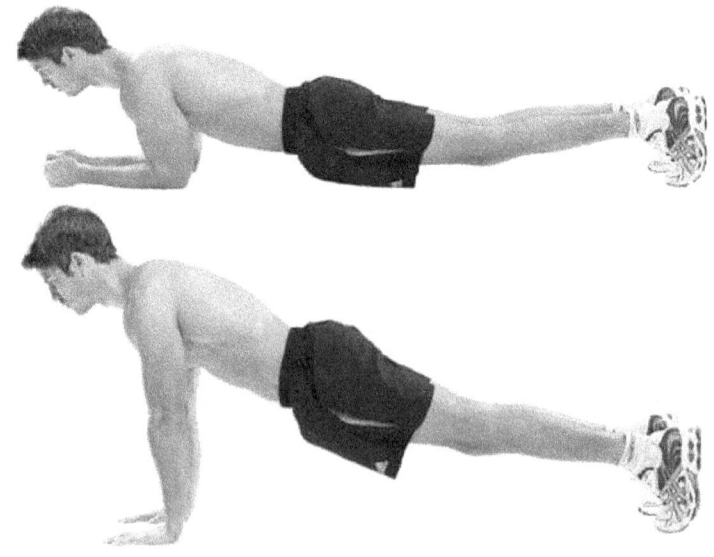

This is another move that looks simple but actually provides an intense full body workout.

Start in plank position (you'll recall this from the beginner's workout at home). Then raise your elbows up off the floor until you are in the downward position of a traditional push up (elbows bent, face right above the floor).

Then, push your elbows back down into plank position. Make sure that your back, butt, and knees are all staying straight (but not locked) throughout this whole process.

One cycle through plank and downward push up position is one repetition. Repeat that cycle 10 times to complete 1 set.

6. *Dynamic Prone Plank (3x20)*

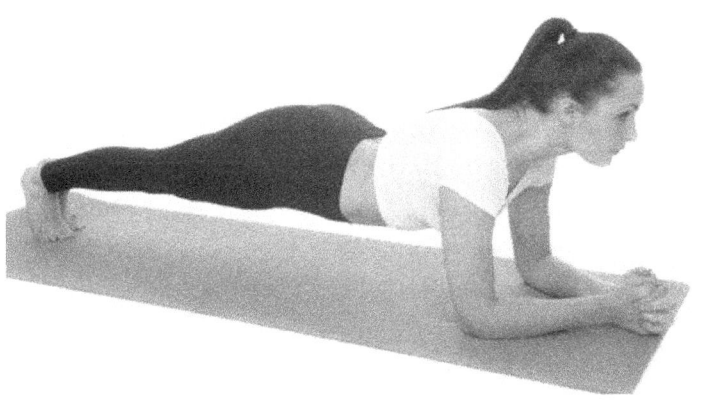

Admittedly, this one looks a little silly but that's what makes it so fun! It also makes it a great workout for your arms, chest, abs, and thighs.

Start in plank position. Then, while keeping everything else straight, raise your hips as high up as you can.

Hold for one breath and then lower back down to a flat plank. Repeat this movement 20 times per set (or more if you can).

If you want more of a cardio workout, take out the one breath pause before lowering back down. Just move up and down continuously.

At the Gym

This is a full body strength-training workout for the gym. Start with whatever interval ratio you can and work your way up to doing 60 seconds of high intensity exercise followed by 30 seconds of low intensity (with no full rest until you've finished the entire workout).

Remember, doing low intensity instead of rest is for more advanced stages so don't start there, work your way up to it. Also, your low intensity intervals should not be more than half of your high intensity exercise.

For weight training, that means use half the weight in half the time. For cardio training - half the resistance (or half the speed) in half the time.

1. Bench Press

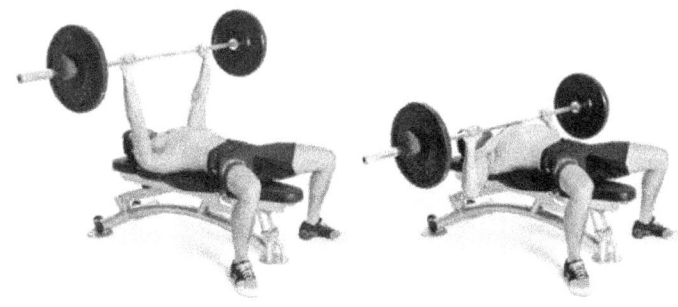

The bench press can seem intimidating but as long as you've got the right weight and someone to spot you, you are safe.

Just make sure your spotter is at least as strong as you are so they can actually lift the bar up if they need to.

Do 5 sets of 10 repetitions at 50% of your 10RM (more on that below).

One repetition is bringing the bar all the way down to your chest without letting any weight onto your chest and then lifting it all the way back up without locking your elbows.

Pay attention to your form more than your speed but go as quickly as you can through the repetitions.

Give yourself 30 to 40 seconds of rest between each set.

2. Leg Press

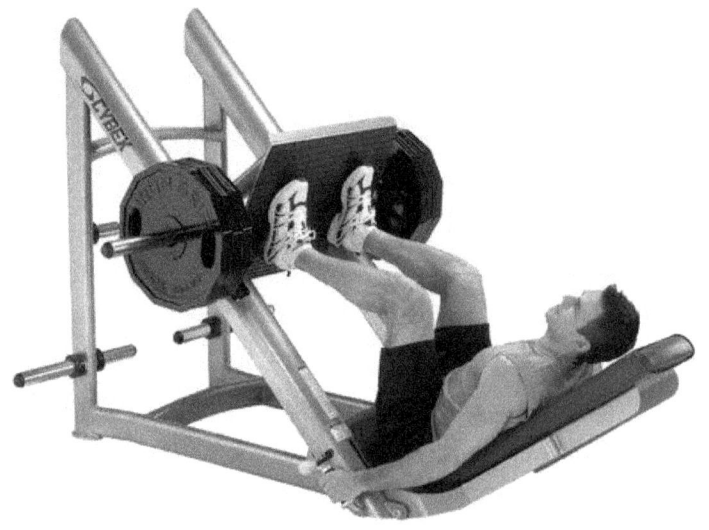

The leg press is done with the machine where you press your feet against a small plate and have to push that plate upward by extending your legs straight.

Do 5 sets of 10 repetitions on this machine using 50% of your 10RM. again, pay attention to your form but go as quickly as you can while still maintaining good form.

Never lock your knees. Take 30 to 40 second rests after finishing each set.

3. Arm Curls

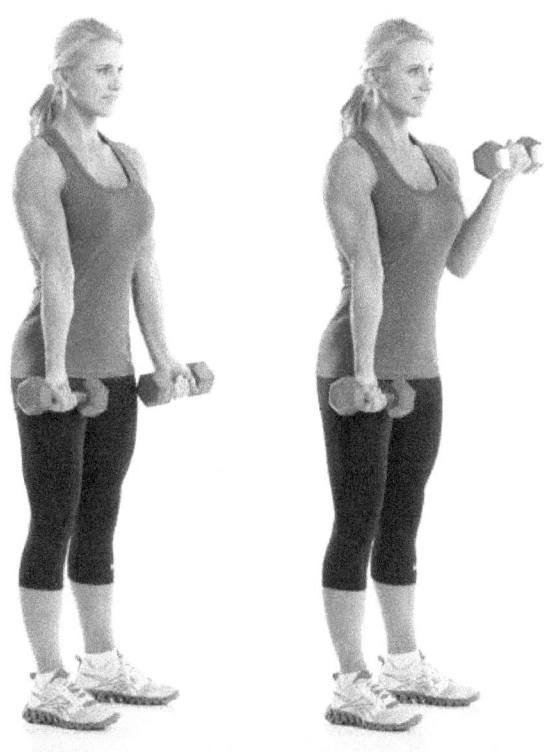

This one is done just with free weights. While standing in a sturdy posture (legs set at a hip width apart), hold a weight (50% of your 10RM) in one hand.

Put your arms straight out in front of you, with elbow slightly bent and the weight facing upward. Put your free hand on your hip for a more secure posture.

While keeping your upper arm straight, bend your elbow and pull the weight toward your shoulder.

Straighten your elbow again. Repeat this 10 times for one set.

Do 5 sets for each arm for 10 sets total. Instead of the rest periods you have been taking in the previous two exercises, just alternate arms to allow each arm to rest while you exercise the other.

4. *Leg Extension*

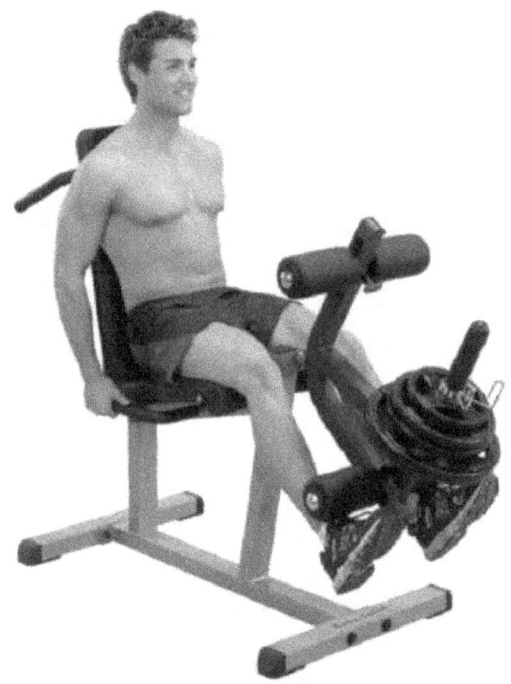

This exercise is done with the machine where you have the bar going across your shins and you need to lift it by lifting your legs and straightening them.

Do 5 sets of 10 repetitions using 50% of your 10RM. Take 30 to 40 seconds to rest between each set.

5. *Wide Grip Pull Down*

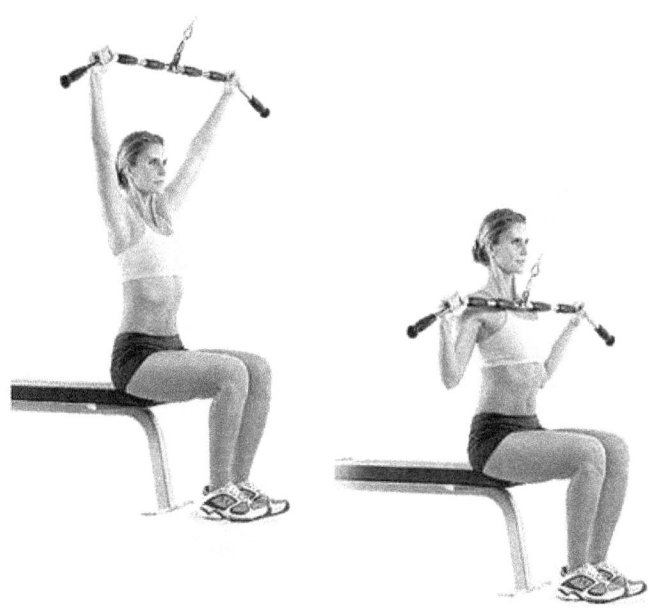

To do this one, you'll use the machine that has the thin bar hanging from a cable, which is attached to a stack of weights (lat pull-down machine).

Set it to the correct weight (50% of your 10RM again). Sit on it so that you are facing away from the stack of weights. Reach up and grip the bar firmly with your palms facing the same direction that you are looking.

Pull the bar down behind your neck and then push it back up. Do not just let the bar fly back up; control its upward movement just as much as you control its downward movement.

For this exercise, you'll want to pay careful attention to form so that you don't slam down on your neck. You don't want the bar to actually touch your neck, just drop down behind it. Use careful, controlled movements but do go as quickly as possible while still maintaining complete control over the machine.

Do 5 sets of 10 repetitions. Take 30 to 40 second rests between each set.

6. *Free Weight Lunges*

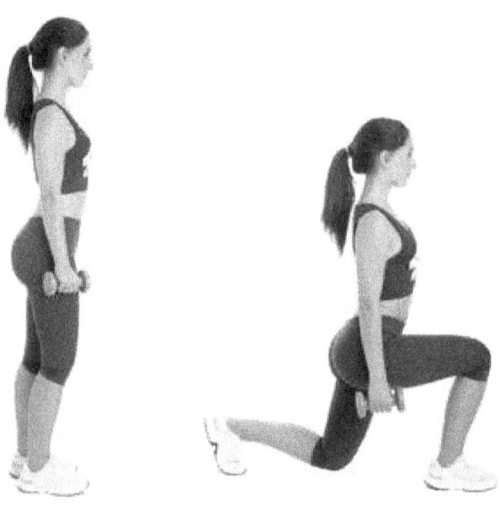

For your last exercise of this workout, you'll go back to the free weights.

This time, you can use the full weight that you can handle because you will just be holding them instead of lifting them.

Now, hold a weight in both hands and let your arms hang by your sides but remember to keep your elbows slightly bent so that they don't lock.

While holding the weights, do lunges on alternating legs. Go as deep into the lunge as possible so that you really feel the stretch in your back leg and the pressure in your front thigh.

Hold each lunge for 30 seconds then stand up and lunge with the other leg forward. Continue doing this until you can't do anymore. Take a 60-second break.

Then, do more free weight lunges until you can't do anymore. Take another 60-second break. Then, for the last time, do free weight lunges until you can't do anymore.

You'll probably do fewer lunges each time but that's ok. Just try to stop it on an even number so that each leg has done the same amount of work.

This workout should last about 20 minutes' total. But the actual length of time depends on how quickly you can (*safely*) move through all the sets. It may be a little more or a little less. The important thing is to complete all the repetitions.

As always, remember to include a 5-minute warm up and a 5-minute cool down. You can do this by doing a brisk walk or light jog on a treadmill or using an elliptical or stationary bike to get your heart pumping but don't wear yourself out.

After your 5-minute cool down, remember to stretch out all your muscles!

Before you start this work out, you'll need to figure out what your current weight limits are, assuming you haven't already been lifting weights. To test your current ability, you'll need to have a pre-workout test day.

Do each of the 6 exercises listed. Put as much weight as you think you can probably lift and do 10 repetitions. If you can't complete 10 repetitions, take off some weight.

If you can do 10 repetitions without feeling at all like you just worked out, it's too light and you need to add more weight. The goal is to find the amount of weight where you can do 10 full repetitions but after those 10, the muscles you were using have burned out.

In weight training lingo, this amount of weight is your 10RM. Write down or otherwise note your 10RM for each of the 6 exercises above.

The next day, you will use 50% of your 10RM. The reason you aren't using your full amount is because you will be doing a lot more than just 10 repetitions during the workout.

If you're enjoying this book and would love to let other potential readers know how great it is, please take a few seconds to leave a review on Amazon.com.

Step 5

Speed Up Your Progress with Muscle Confusion

In step 5, you will learn the science behind muscle confusion and how incorporating it into your workout routine can help you burn fat as fast as possible.

After you read about muscle confusion and how it works, you'll get another 4 sample workouts (2 at the beginner level and 2 at the intermediate level) that you can combine with the workouts you chose from the previous two chapters to create a well-rounded workout plan that combines all the benefits of cardio exercise, strength training, *and* muscle confusion for the ultimate fat blasting routine that will have you burning calories up to 300% faster than your old routine.

What Is Muscle Confusion?

Muscle confusion is the practice of changing your training program to keep your muscles guessing. The idea is that your body eventually hits a plateau if you keep doing the same exact exercises with the same number of repetitions every single time you work out.

By changing certain parts of your workout, your muscles cannot adapt or predict what it will have to do. When the workout is unpredictable, your muscles are constantly challenged to perform and push past their own limits.

There are many different variables of your workout that you can change in order to keep your body from adapting and stagnating.

Here are 5 of the variables that you can regularly change up to maintain unpredictability.

Exercise variation

Change the type of exercise you do in your workout but replace it with the same kind of exercise.

For example, if you want to vary your resistance cardio workout, hop on the stationary bike or take a dip in the pool instead of going on the treadmill.

If you are trying to vary your weight training routine, use a different kind of machine that targets similar muscle groups or opt for an equipment free exercise that targets the same muscle groups you were working on with weights.

For the muscle confusion workouts below, find different yoga poses that stretch or work on the same muscles or find new exercises to target your neglected muscles.

Pauses

In addition to changing the type of exercise you do, you can change the length of your rests. This is something you will naturally do with your HIIT workout plan because as you improve, the pauses will grow shorter at the same time that your high intensity intervals grow longer. This is yet another benefit of HIIT.

Muscle confusion is already programmed right into it since you will continue to change the length of your high intensity and low intensity intervals. But you can also do this within a single workout.

If your first intervals are 20 seconds of high intensity and 40 seconds of low intensity; then your next intervals can be something like 25 seconds of high intensity and 35 seconds of low intensity.

Switch around within one workout to achieve even more muscle confusion and progress faster.

Continuous tension

This variable is related to pauses. Within one set of repetitions, you tend to briefly pause between movements.

For example, if you are doing lunges, you tend to pause for a brief couple seconds between each lunge when you are back in the standing position. With continuous tension, you eliminate those small pauses.

Rather than stopping in the standing position, your next leg will already be moving into a lunge even as your first leg is still coming back.

Don't use continuous tension in every single workout session; but add it in a few times here and there. If you are doing 5 sets of repetitions, you can do one set using continuous tension. Alternatively, pick one day from each week where you do all sets with continuous tension.

This variable does not apply to resistance cardio since cardio already includes it (unless for some reason you are pausing to stand between each step when you run!).

Partial repetitions

Another way to change up your strength training or muscle confusion routine is to change the number of repetitions. If you normally do 10 repetitions per set, change some sets to 5 repetitions and others to 15.

With the yoga routines below, try taking out one or two moves and then do the other ones more than you normally do. Another way to do partial repetitions is to shrink each repetition.

For example, if you're on the bench press, only take the bar halfway down instead of bringing it all the way to your chest. You can even alternate within one set.

For the first repetition, go through the full range of the move. For the second repetition, only go halfway. Continue alternating in this pattern for the full set or even for all the sets that you do.

Super sets

This is an extreme version of changing the length of pauses between sets in the sense that you eliminate all the pauses.

For each exercise, complete all the sets as if it was one long "super" set. You can then take a regular sized pause before switching to the next exercise or you can go for the gold and turn your entire workout session into the most super of super sets!

Just remember to be careful. This is definitely not something you should try on your first trip to the gym. Save it for after you've had a few weeks to build up some muscle and skill.

The workouts below can be done as they are written for the first 4 weeks or so. After that, change it up by altering the different variables that you have just read about above.

Do this with each of the workouts in your workout plan. In your resistance cardio routine, for example, you can change what cardio activity you do every month. For the first month, you can run. Then, try swimming the next month.

For the strength training workouts from step 4, you can change the order you do the exercises in and change the number of repetitions or the length of pauses between sets and so on.

Keep changing it up every 4 weeks. This will give you enough time for you to really progress with a certain routine without allowing your body the time to hit a plateau and stop progressing.

Beginner Workouts for Muscle Confusion

HIIT Yoga workout

Below is a series of 10 high intensity interval moves using yoga poses. You will need to set a timer for 20 seconds and repeat the move as many times as possible in that 20 seconds.

Between each high intensity interval, rest in child's pose, mountain pose, or reclined mountain (descriptions to follow). Your rest pose can be whatever is most comfortable. Just remain in it for 40 seconds before moving on to the next high intensity interval sequence.

Before you start, do a short warm up to warm your muscles up and increase flexibility.

Here is a sample warm up sequence you can follow:

Begin in mountain pose. This is where you stand straight and tall with your arms raised straight up over your head and your palms parallel, facing each other.

Hold this pose and take 5 long, slow, deep breaths. Fill your entire chest with your breath and slowly release it.

As you exhale on your 5th breath, bend down at the waist to touch the floor. Keep your legs straight. This pose is forward bend.

If you can't touch the floor while keeping your legs straight, hold on to your ankles or shins. Take 3 deep breaths while remaining in forward bend.

As you exhale the 3rd breath, place your palms on the floor and jump your legs back into downward dog. This pose is when you are making an upside-down V shape with your body.

Your arms, back, and legs are straight, your hips are high in the air, and your heels are on the ground (or as close to the ground as you can get them). Hold this pose for 5 deep breaths.

As you breathe, continue to push your heels and palms toward the floor. Don't let your shoulders are back bend. The weight of your body should be fully placed on your hands and feet.

As you exhale the 5th breath, move down into plank pose. This is like the downward position of a push up.

Your body is straight like a plank; your toes are the only part of your feet that are touching the floor; and your arms are bent down so that you are hovering just above the floor. Inhale deeply while in plank pose, as you exhale, move up into upward facing dog.

Upward facing dog is when your legs are on the floor; the tops of your feet are flat against the floor; your torso is lifted up; and your arms are straight with palms pressed into the floor. It is almost as if you are attempting to fold yourself in half backwards. Hold this for 2 deep breaths.

As you exhale the 2nd breath, move back into downward dog. Hold this for 5 deep breaths. Then, on the exhale of the 5th breath; jump back up into forward bend. Hold this for 3 deep breaths. Exhale and slowly rise up into mountain.

Clasp your hands together while they are raised above your head. Pull your arms, shoulders and upper back down and backwards until you feel the muscles in your abdomen stretch.

Hold this for one deep breath. Come back up.

Now, pull your left hand with your right arm and bend to the right until you feel the muscles on your left side stretch. Hold this for one deep breath.

Come back up.

Repeat on the other side. Do each of these stretches one more time.

Now you are ready to start your HIIT yoga workout! (Remember your 40-second rest intervals between each one).

1. ***Chair to Mountain***

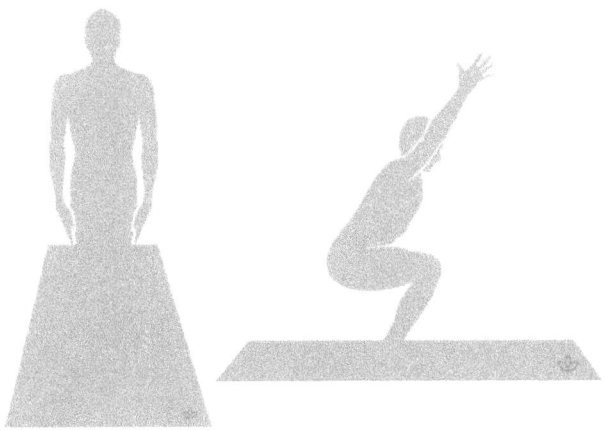

For this one, you will begin in chair pose. To get into chair pose, start in mountain pose. Spread your legs to hip width apart.

Bend down as if you are about to take a seat. Lean your torso forward. Your hands should remain raised above your head as they are with mountain pose.

From chair pose, raise back up into mountain. Inhales as you raise up into mountain, exhale as you sink down into chair pose. Rapidly repeat this cycle of moving from chair pose to mountain pose for the entirety of your high intensity interval.

Focus on your breathing and your form.

2. *Forward Bend with Arm Lifts*

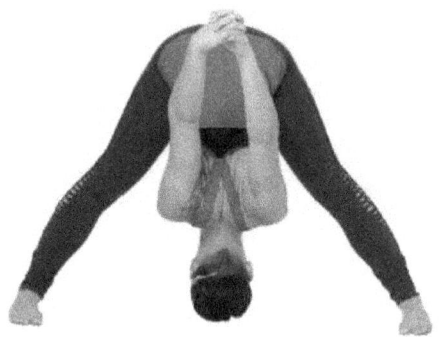

In this sequence you will bend down into a forward bend (description above in the warm up). Rather than touch the floor, clasp your hands together behind your back, and keep your elbows straight.

Now, pull your arms as far out and away from your back as you can and then push them back toward your back. Inhale as you push them toward your back and exhale as you pull them away.

Repeat this movement rapidly for the full high intensity interval. Remember to keep your legs and arms straight. Remain as deeply in forward bend as your flexibility allows you to go.

If you can touch your nose to your thighs, that is what you should be doing this entire time.

3. Lunges, Alternating Legs

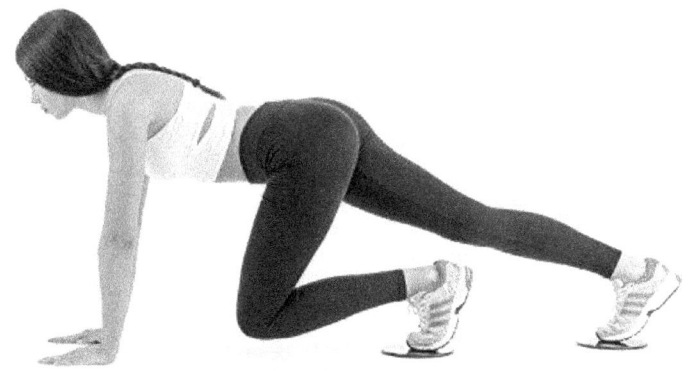

Go into a lunge position. Your front knee should be sitting directly above your ankle so that your shin forms a straight line perpendicular to the ground.

Your back knee should be straight and your back toes should be the only part of your foot that is touching the floor. You'll feel a stretch in the top of your back leg. Put your palms down flat on the floor.

They should be in line with your foot and positioned just wider than shoulder width apart. With your arms in position, jump your back leg up and your front leg back so that you are again lunging but with your legs switched.

Keep your arms straight and palms on the floor the entire time. Inhale on one jump and exhale on the other. Continue alternating your legs as quickly as possible for the full high intensity interval.

4. *Downward Dog with Leg Movements*

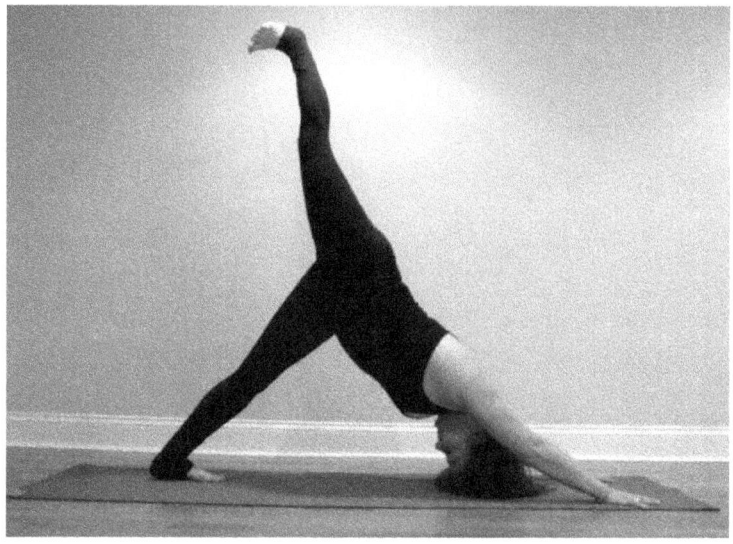

Get into downward dog (description can be found above in the warm up section). While maintaining a perfect and balanced form in this position, raise one leg up behind you as high in the air as you can while keeping the knee straight.

Now swing it down, bend the knee and pull the leg under and in toward your chest. Then place it back down in its original position. Repeat with the other leg.

Continue doing this sequence of movements with each of your legs for the full length of your high intensity interval.

5. *Downward Dog with Arm Movements*

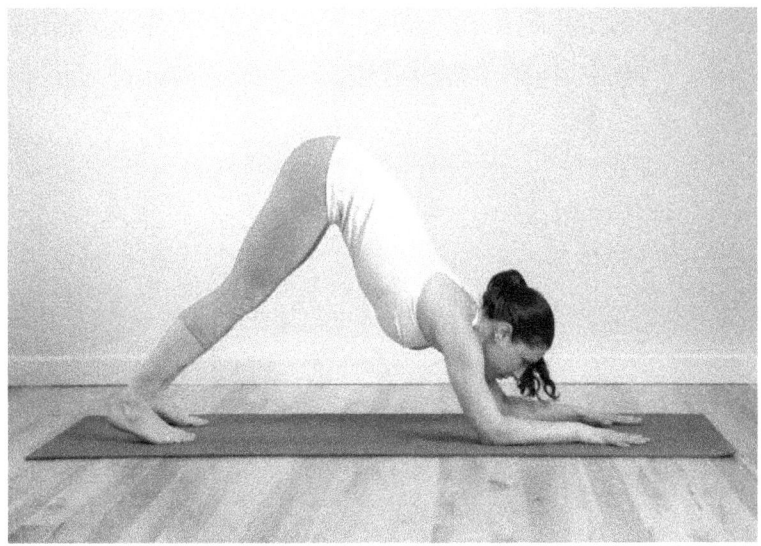

Return to downward dog position. Instead of your legs, you're going to work on your arms this time.

Bend one arm down so that elbow is resting on the floor while maintaining the rest of your downward dog pose as it should be.

Bend the other arm down. Raise the arm you bent first and follow it with your other arm.

Now repeat but start with the opposite arm that you started with the first time. Continue to bend your arms down and raise them back up for your full high intensity interval. Be sure to maintain the downward dog pose.

With this sequence, it can be easy to start letting your back bend or your knees sink down. Keep them straight throughout the movements. It should be only your arms that move.

6. *Plank with Leg Lifts*

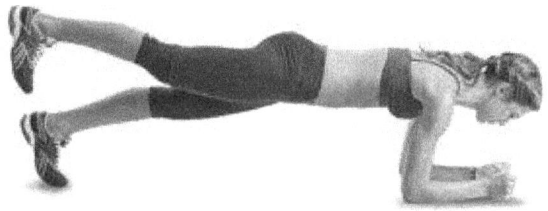

Get down into plank pose (you can find the description above in the warm up section). Instead of having your arms bent, however, keep them straight as if you are in the upward position of a push up.

Hold this pose and lift one leg up as high as you can without bending the knee. Lower it back down. Repeat with the other leg.

Continue to raise alternate legs for the duration of your high intensity interval.

7. Reclined Mountain to Seated Forward Bend

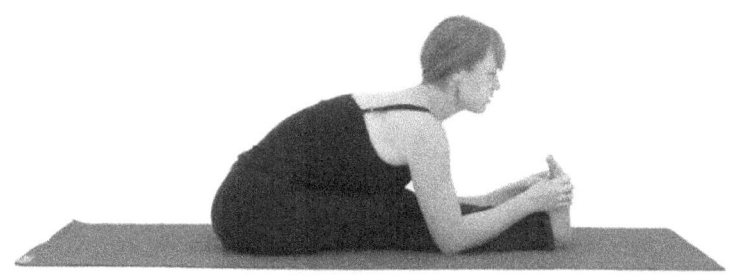

Get into reclined mountain pose. This looks similar to mountain pose except that you are lying down on the floor instead of standing up. Your arms should, again, be raised above your head. From this position, sit up using only your torso. Do not use your arms to hoist yourself up.

Instead of sitting, fold all the way down into seated forward bend. This is similar to a regular forward bend except that you are sitting down.

Clasp your hands around your feet. If you cannot reach your feet without bending your knees, clasp your hands around your ankles or shins (however far down you can go without bending your knees).

Once you have done that, lift out of seated forward bend and lower back down into reclined mountain. The power to move yourself should be coming entirely from your torso. Do not use your arms to push yourself up.

Continue to move from reclined mountain into seated forward bend and back again as rapidly as you can for your high intensity interval.

8. *Seated to Camel Pose*

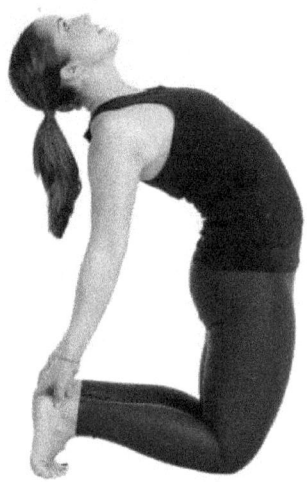

Start this pose by sitting on top of your shins with the tops of your feet pressed into the floor. Your back should be straight and your hands should be resting on your thighs.

Once seated, lift your hips up so that you are standing on your knees. Bend backwards and grab each ankle with each hand. This is camel pose.

Let go of your ankles and raise back out of camel pose. Come back to a seated position. Repeat this sequence of movement as rapidly as possible for your high intensity interval.

9. *Chair to Forward Bend*

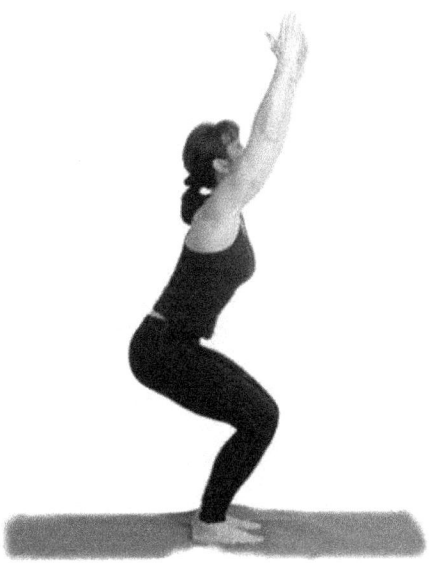

You will remember chair pose from the first position you did of this HIIT yoga workout (when you were moving from chair into mountain).

Get back into chair pose. This time, however, you'll fold down into forward bend instead of raising up into mountain. Do this by lowering your torso and arms to place your palms on the floor while straightening your legs and raising your hips.

Try to keep your arms and torso in line as if they are one solid piece throughout this movement. Continue moving through chair pose into a forward bend and back again as quickly as you can for your high intensity interval.

10. *Proud Warrior with Rotations*

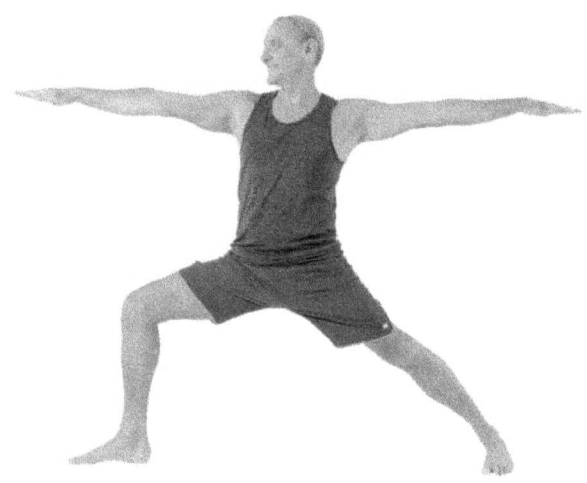

In this final sequence, you will start in proud warrior. Your legs will be in a lunge position.

Your back foot should be flat against the ground and turned slightly to the side while your front foot points straight as it normally does. Feel the stretch in your back leg.

Raise your arms out to the sides so that you are forming a T shape with your upper body. Your palms should be flat, facing the floor. Look out at the tip of your front hand.

Bend your torso pack without moving your legs or arms and clasp your back shin or ankle with your back hand.

Raise your front arm up as you do this. Then unclasp and come back to proud warrior position.

This time, bend your torso forward (again without moving any other part of you) and place your front palm on the floor just beside the outside of your foot.

Bring your back arm up and shoot it above your head, palm facing the floor until you feel the stretch in your side. Move fluidly and quickly through these 3 separate positions for your high intensity interval.

Repeat this entire sequence of 3 poses again with your alternate leg forward this time.

After you have completed all of your movements for the HIIT yoga workout, you'll want to do a cool down to help keep your muscles from tearing or tightening.

For the beginner workout, you can end with the following cool down sequence:

After finishing the proud warrior with rotations sequence, place both palms on the floor, in line with your front leg.

Bring your front leg back and go into downward dog. Hold this for 5 deep breaths.

As you exhale the last breath, move down into plank pose (arms bent). Hold this for one deep breath.

As you exhale, move into upward dog. Hold this for 2 deep breaths.

From upward dog, bend back into child's pose.

For child's pose, your legs will be as they are in seated position (from the 8th yoga sequence you did above).

Instead of sitting upright, however, your torso will be bent over your legs; your arms raised above your head, resting on the floor with palms down; and your forehead will either be on the floor so that you are staring at the ground or you can turn your head to the side and place your cheek on the ground (whichever is more comfortable for you).

Essentially, you are in the fetal position but facing the ground instead of laying on your side.

While in child's pose, take 10 long, deep breaths. Allow yourself to release the tension from your back, neck, and arms.

Push all the stress away and take a moment to deeply relax. As you exhale that 10th breath, sit up and then lay back in reclined mountain.

Allow the tension in your legs, stomach, chest and everywhere else to release.

From reclined mountain, rise up to a sitting position with your legs straight out in front of you. Reach down and grab one foot, pull your foot up as you bend your leg.

Press the sole of your foot to your upper thigh so that your bent leg is lying flat on the floor to the side. Reach down and clasp your hands around your other foot.

Keep your knee straight. If you can't clasp your foot while keeping your knee straight, hold on to your ankle or shin.

Hold this position for 5 deep breaths. Then, lift out of it, straighten your bent leg and repeat this same movement with your other leg.

Hold it again for 5 deep breaths.

When you have come back up to sitting position with your legs still straight out in front of you; pull one leg up again but this time place the foot on the floor on the other side of your straight leg.

Hug your knee to your chest with one arm and twist your back to look behind you. Hold this for 5 deep breaths. Put your leg back and repeat this with the other side. Hold again for 5 deep breaths.

Straighten your legs again and then lie back down into reclined mountain pose. Relax and feel proud that you made it through to the end of your workout.

Remain in this position as long as you like. Then, get up and high five yourself (if your arms are still working)!

Most Neglected Muscles Workout

1. *Resistance Band Side Shuffle*

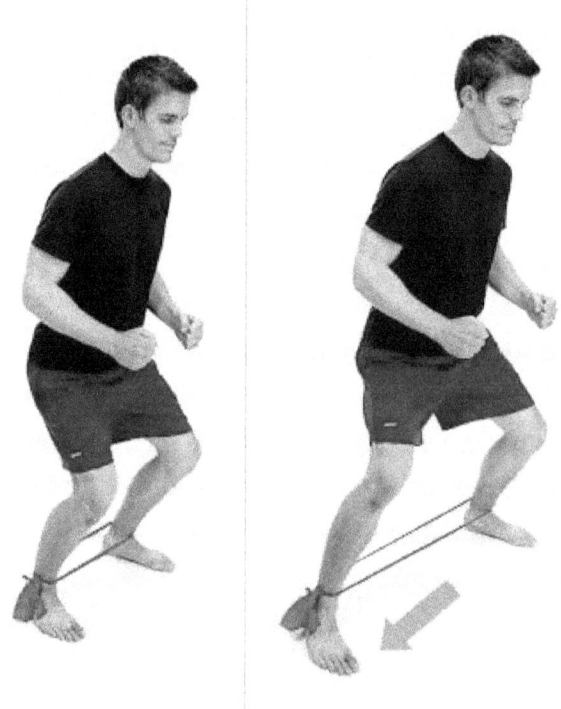

This is just like the side shuffle you read about in step 4 but this time, you will have a small resistance band wrapped around your shins.

Do as many side shuffles as you can during your high intensity interval time. Rest and side shuffle in the other direction for your next high intensity interval.

2. Chest Dips

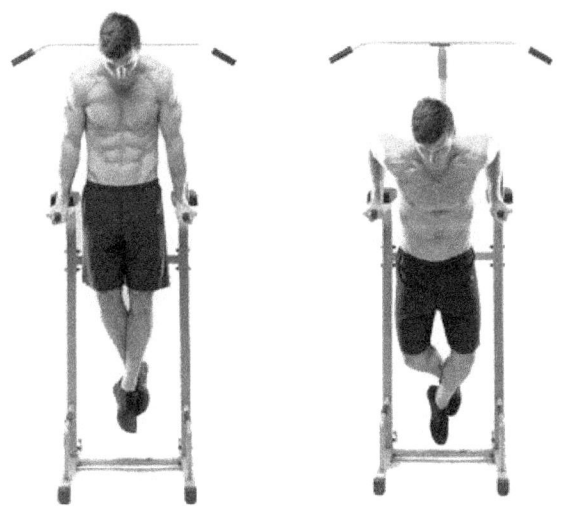

Chest dips require two stable bars that you can grab onto. Bend your legs up so that your arms are carrying your full weight. Raise yourself up and down as many times as you can during your high intensity interval.

3. Reclined Back Extensions

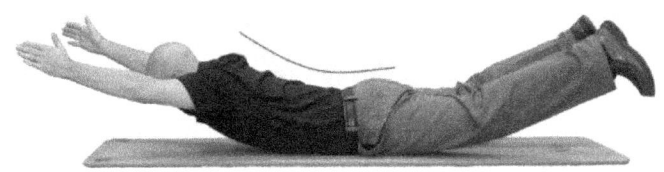

Lay flat on your stomach with your arms above your head and your legs straight.

Raise your arms, head, neck, shoulders, and legs off the floor all at the same time. You'll look sort of like an archery bow without the string.

Your full body weight will be on your lower stomach. Instead of moving in and out of this position, just hold it for the full length of your high intensity interval.

4. Crunches

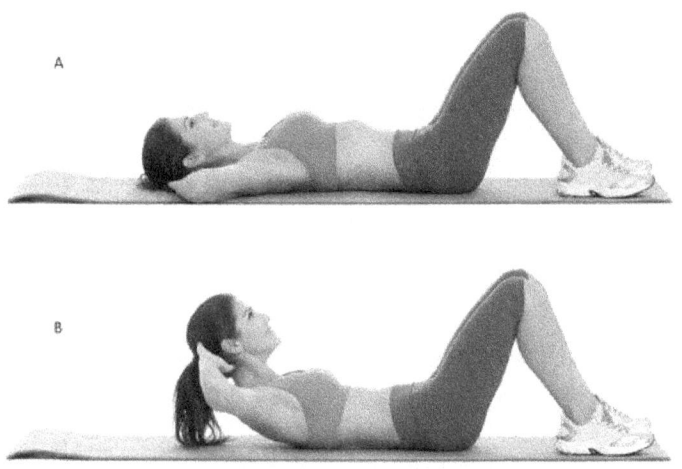

You probably know what crunches are. You can also do sit ups instead if you prefer them. The difference is that sit-ups require you to go all the way up.

Crunches just mean you raise your upper back off the ground. Do as many crunches (or sit ups) as you can for your high intensity interval.

5. *Single Leg Hip Thrusts*

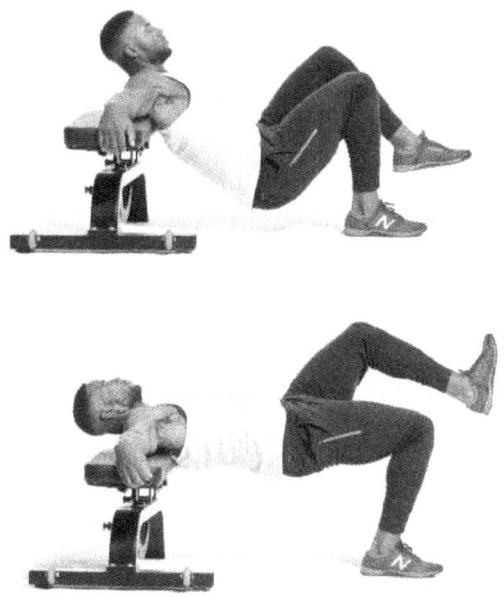

Lean back on a bench with your elbows. Plant your feet a little wider than hip width apart. The rest of your body should be free aside from your forearms and the bottom of your feet.

Extend one leg out in front of you (knee straight). Raise your hips up so that you form a kind of bridge. Lower back down.

Repeat this for your high intensity interval. Take your rest period and then do the same thing with the other leg raised.

6. *Rotational Skater Jump*

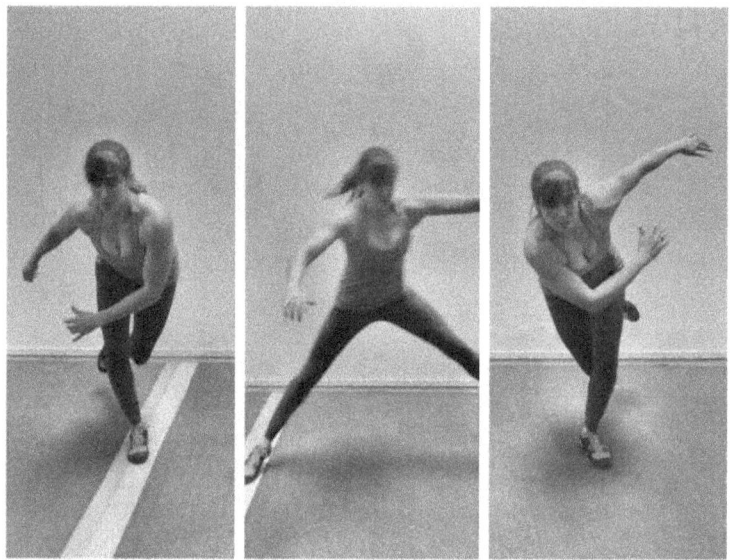

Stand up with your legs slightly wider than hip width apart. Bend your knees slightly and bend your torso down.

Your elbows should be bent and your hands closed in a fist. It should look like you are on a set of skis holding ski poles. Lift one leg off the ground and twist your torso to the other side.

As you lower that leg to the ground, lift the other leg off the ground and twist to the opposite side.

It will look like you are ice skating in place. (I know, you started as a skier and now suddenly you're an ice skater. It's OK; we're using our imagination, here!).

Repeat this process for your final high intensity interval.

Intermediate Workouts for Muscle Confusion

HIIT Yoga Workout

Below is a series of 10 high intensity interval moves using yoga poses. You will need to set a timer for 30 seconds and repeat the move as many times as possible in that 30 seconds.

Between each high intensity interval, rest in child's pose, mountain pose, or reclined mountain (descriptions above). Your rest pose can be whatever is most comfortable.

Just remain in it for 30 seconds before moving on to the next high intensity interval sequence.

Before you start working through each of these movements, do a short warm up to get your muscles warm and increase flexibility. You can use the same warm up sequence described above for the beginner's HIIT yoga workout routine.

After you've completed that, you are ready to start your HIIT Yoga Workout (Remember your 30-second rest intervals between each one)!

1. Chair to One Leg Extended Pose

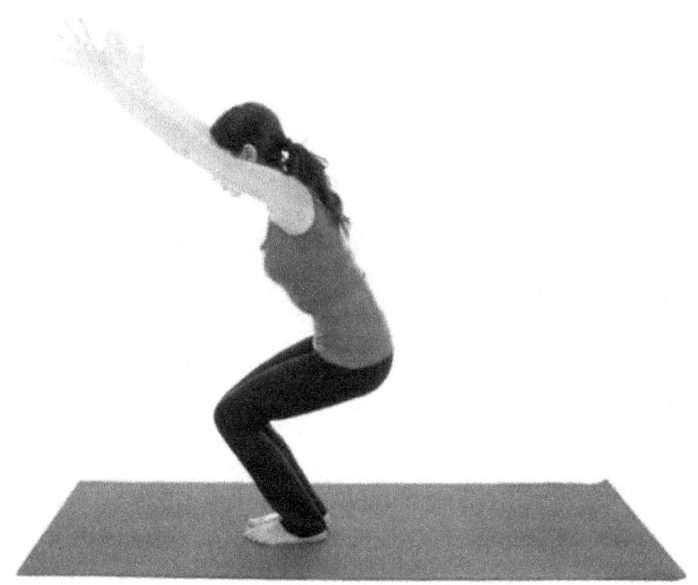

For this sequence, you will begin in chair pose (you can find a detailed description of this in the beginner's HIIT yoga workout routine).

While keeping both knees bent and both arms raised as they should be, lift one leg out and up to extend it straight in front of you as high up as you can without falling over.

Try not to move any other part of your body except for this leg. Lower back down and repeat with the other leg. Continue rapidly raising alternate legs while holding chair pose the entire time for your first high intensity interval.

2. Mountain with Arms Raised to Lunge, Alternating Legs

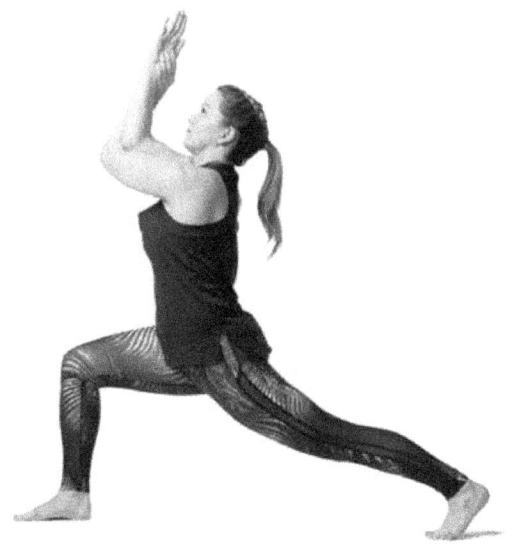

Begin in mountain pose (you can find a description of this pose in the warm up sequence in the beginner's HIIT yoga workout).

Keep your arms raised and your torso straight as you jump one leg back and one leg forward and sink into a deep lunge.

Then, jump up and stand in mountain pose again. When you jump back into a lunge again, make sure that the opposite leg is in front this time.

Remember to keep your torso and arms straight the whole time. The only movement should be in your legs.

Repeat this sequence (remembering to alternate legs) for the full duration of your high intensity interval.

3. *Wide Leg Stretch with Forward Bends*

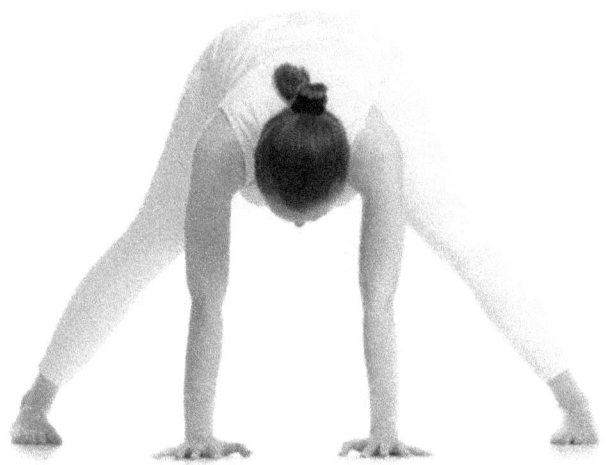

For this, you will need to get into a wide leg stretch. Start in mountain pose. Put your hands on your hips.

Jump your legs out to the side about 3 feet apart.

Spread them a little further if you can. You want to feel the stretch in your inner thighs. Keep your hands on your hips and bend forward to look at the floor.

Bend until your torso is parallel with the ground. Then raise back up. The only movement should be your torso bending up and down.

Keep your feet firmly planted on the floor and your knees straight. Your back should also remain straight, do not allow your back to bend.

Use your hips to bend your torso up and down. Repeat this as quickly as possible (without falling over or losing form) until your high interval time is up.

4. *Deep Lunge to Exalted Warrior to Brave Warrior, Alternating Sides*

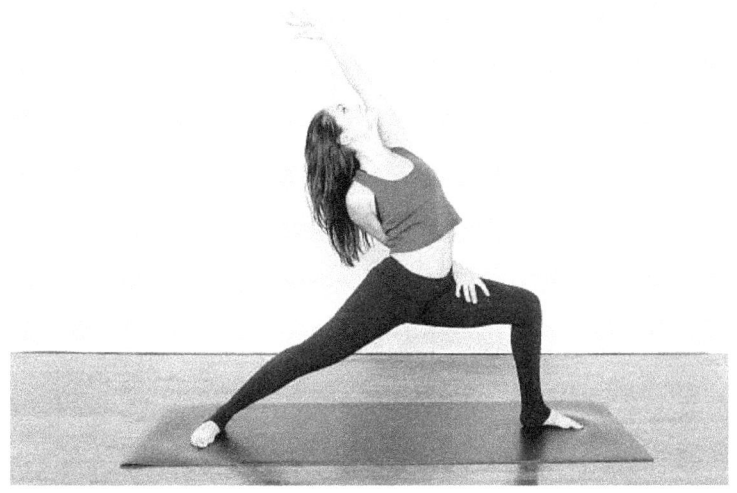

This sequence begins in a deep lunge with your back knee lightly resting on the floor (be careful not to actually put any pressure on your back knee).

Using only the strength of your legs, raise out of this lunge into a normal lunge. Raise your arms above your head (as if this was mountain pose).

Then, raise your back leg off the ground and pull yourself forward so that you are balancing entirely on your front leg (which should be mostly straight with a slight bend).

Your body should form a straight line from the tips of your fingers to the toe of your raised foot. You will look like a T with a very long upper part.

Carefully lower your leg back down, return to exalted warrior. Then, return to the deep lunge. Continue moving through these 3 positions for your full high intensity interval. Repeat this again with your alternate leg forward this time.

5. *Plank with Arm and Leg Lifts*

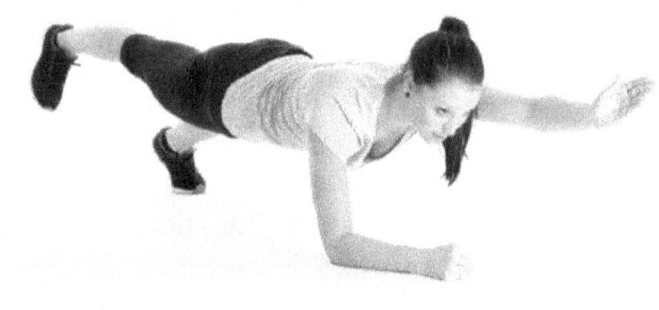

Get into plank pose (description in the warm up sequence from the beginner's HIIT yoga workout). Keep your arms straight instead of bending them as you usually would for this pose.

Once in position, bend your elbows to do a push up. After you come up, raise your left arm up and straight in front of you. At the same time, raise your right leg up and straight back.

Put them down.

Do another push up.

When you come back up this time, you will raise your right arm and your left leg. Continue through this sequence (alternating the arms and legs that you lift) for the full length of your high intensity interval.

6. *Plank with Side Jumps*

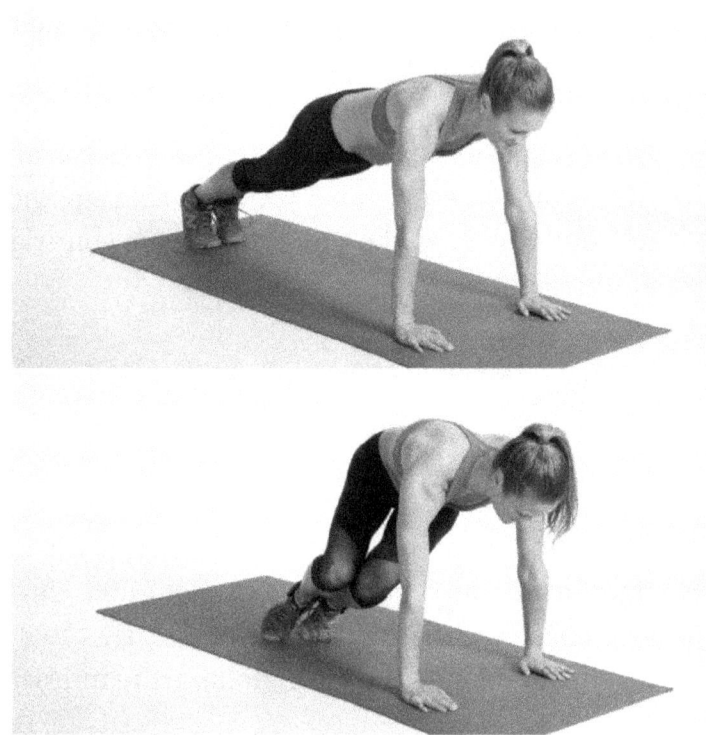

Return to plank pose (with your arms bent). However, if you find that you cannot do this with your arms bent, you can modify it by doing it with your arms straight.

From plank position, jump both legs about 6 inches to the left side. Then jump them about 6 inches to your right side. Keep your legs glued together and do not let your knees bend.

The power of this movement should be coming from your abs, hips, and thighs.

Continue jumping from side to side throughout your high intensity interval.

7. Plank to Forward Bend

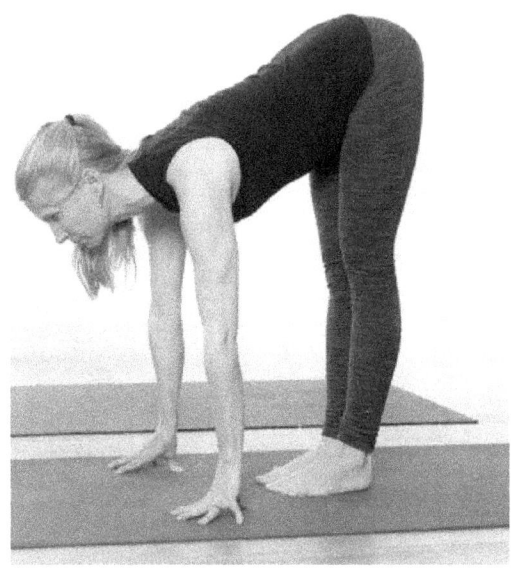

You're going to get into plank position again. Keep your arms straight for this one. Once in position, jump your legs forward and come into a forward bend.

Then, jump pack into plank position. Continue this is as a fluid and quick movement for your entire high intensity interval.

8. Rocking Bow Pose

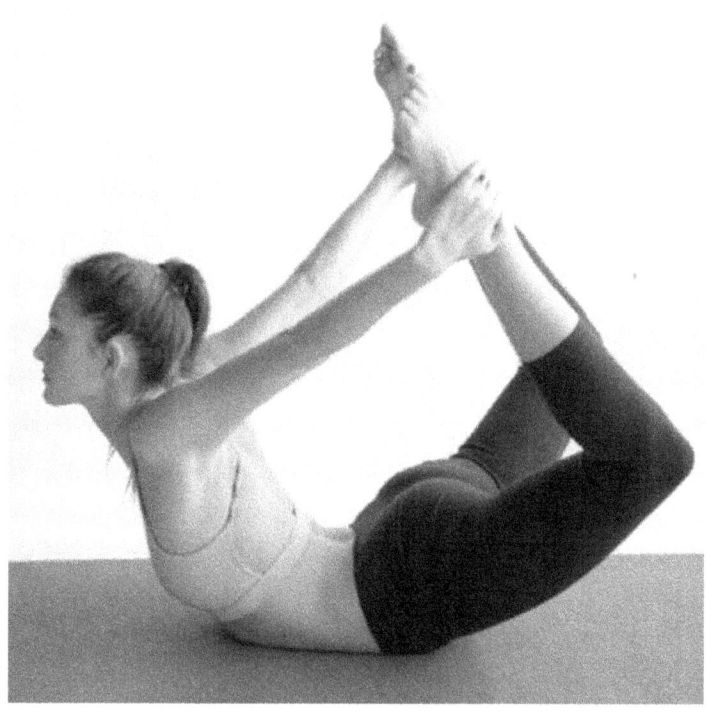

Lay down flat on your stomach. Bend your legs up so that you are kicking your butt. Grab an ankle with each hand.

Raise your legs and arms upward so that you are balanced only on your lower stomach. Use your chest and shoulders to rock yourself forward.

Use your shins to rock yourself back. Keep your hands clasped around your ankles and keep yourself raised up off the ground the entire time.

Continue to rock from front to back on your stomach until your high intensity interval time is up.

9. Side Plank with Knee Lifts

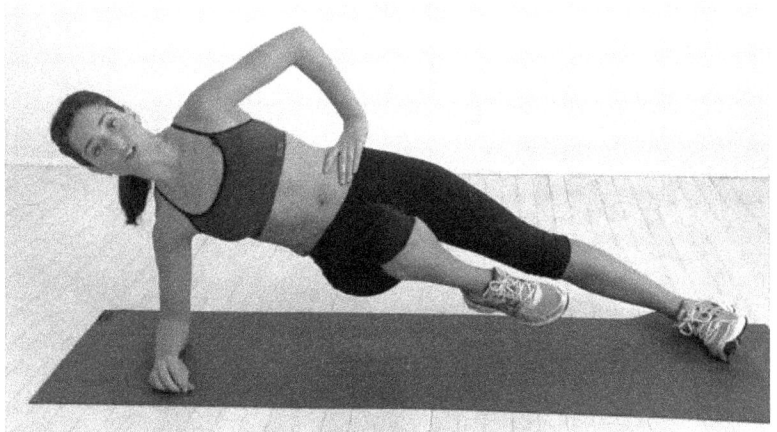

Begin in plank pose with your arms straight. Lift one arm up and stick straight out to the side.

Raise yourself up so that you are balancing on one arm and the outside of one foot.

Rest your top leg on your bottom leg so that your torso and legs form a straight line.

Bend your free arm down and gently place your palm on the back of your head. Lift your top leg and bend your knee into your chest. At the same time, you will bend your elbow down to meet your knee.

Release the leg back down and raise your elbow back up. This is sort of like you are doing half a crunch while holding yourself up.

Repeat this sequence for your full high intensity interval. Take your rest period and then repeat this one again on your other side.

10. *Half Moon with Knee Lifts*

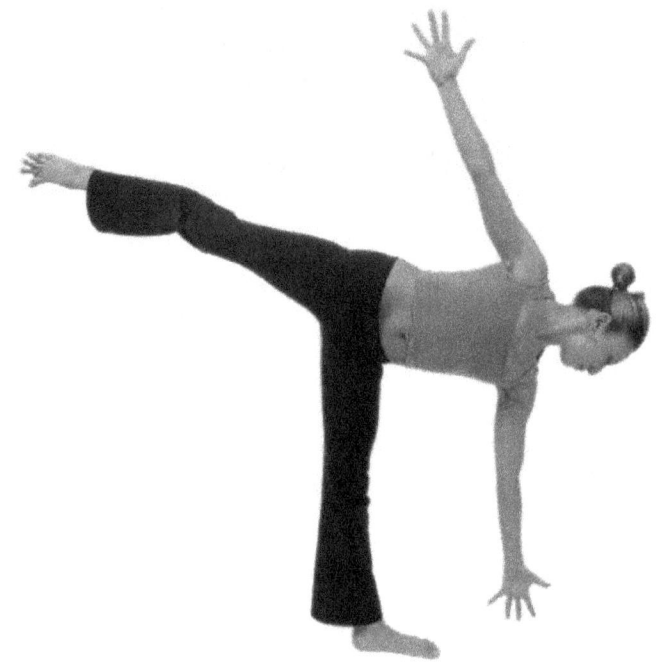

To get into half-moon pose, begin in proud warrior (description can be found in the 10 sequence of the beginner HIIT yoga workout).

Then, lift your back leg off the floor as you straighten out your front leg. Place your palms on the floor.

While holding this pose, pull your back knee up to your chest and come up to a one legged standing position, hugging your knee to your chest.

Release the knee and move back into the half-moon pose. Repeat this as quickly as you can without losing balance for your full high intensity interval.

Use your rest period and then repeat this again on your other side.

Once you have completed all the movements, remember to do a short cool down. This will prevent injury and give you time to catch your breath again before you get on with your day.

You can use the same cool down sequence from the beginner's HIIT yoga workout routine.

Most Neglected Muscles Workout

1. *Bent Over Free Weight Lifts*

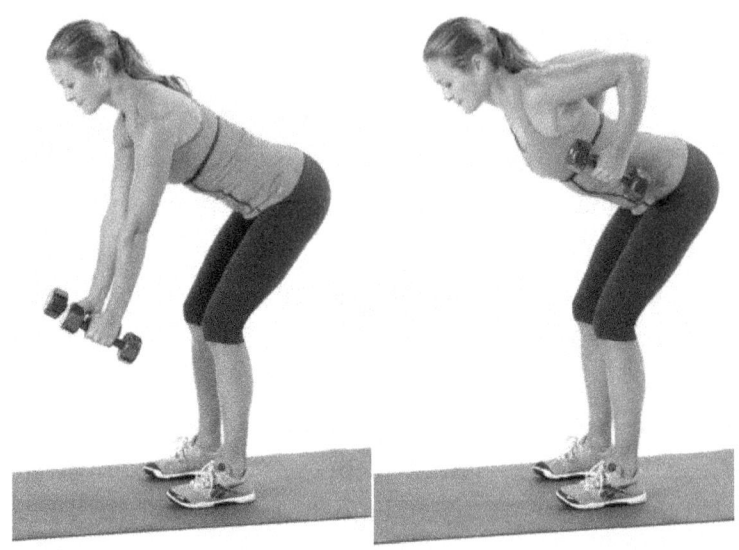

Hold weights in each hand. Stand with your legs hip width apart.

Bend over at the hips, keeping your back straight. Lift both arms up at the same time bending your elbows straight up behind you (as if you are a bird with wings raised).

Continue to raise and lower the weights in this way while staying bent over for your first high intensity interval.

2. *Weighted V Ups*

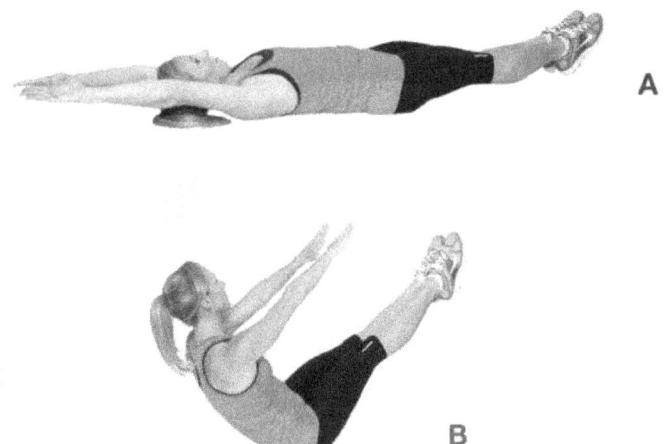

Attach ankle weights to your ankles. Hold light weights in each hand. Lie down with your legs straight and your arms straight above you (palms upward).

Raise your legs, arms, and torso upward altogether. Keep everything straight so that you form a V shape. Lower back down.

Repeat this for your full high intensity interval.

3. *Single Leg Hip Thrusts*

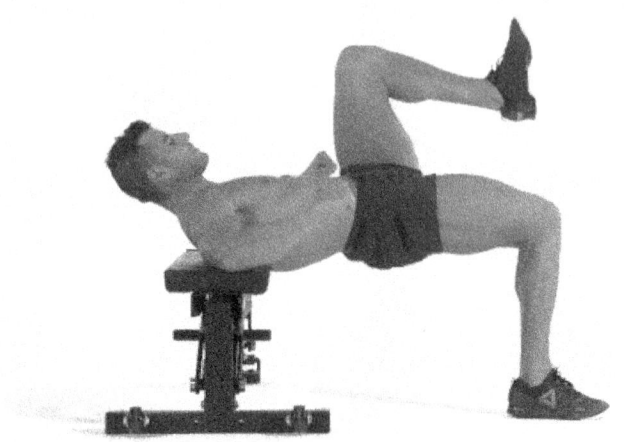

You can find a description of this in the beginner's workout for the most neglected muscles workout. Kick it up a notch by adding ankle weights to your ankles.

4. Reclined Triceps Extensions

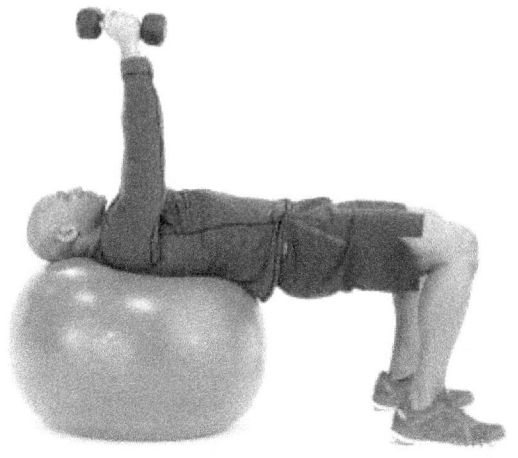

Hold one weight with both hands. Lay back on a large exercise ball. Raise the weight above your head. Allow your elbows to bend.

Pull it back in front of your chest. Move it back above your head. Repeat this for your full high intensity interval.

5. *Weighted Punches*

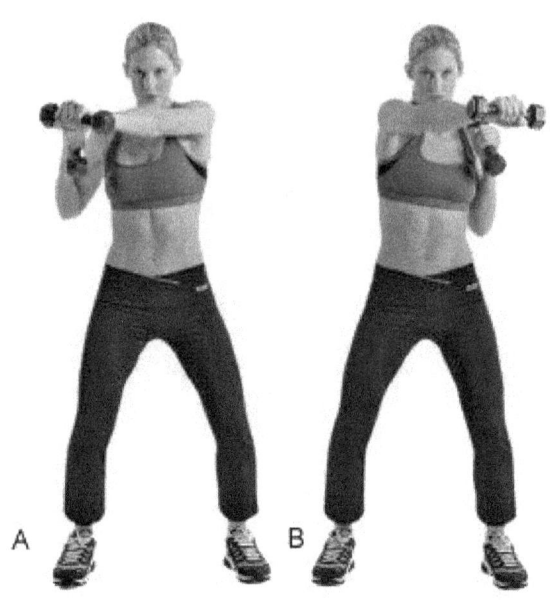

Lay back on the exercise ball again. This time, you should be holding weights in both hands.

Keep your arms out to the side and elbows bent as if you are about to hug someone.

Straighten one arm as you punch it directly above you. As you bring that arm down, punch the other one up. Repeat this for your high intensity interval.

6. *Rotational Skater Jump with Free Weights*

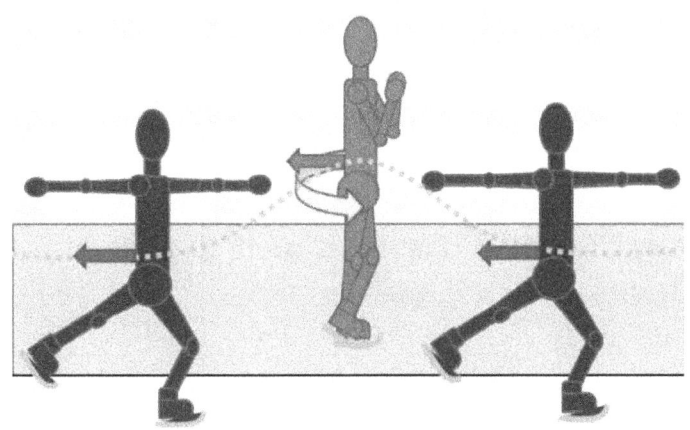

You can find the description of this exercise in the beginner's version of this workout. To kick it up another level, hold weights in your hands while you do it.

7. Chest Dips

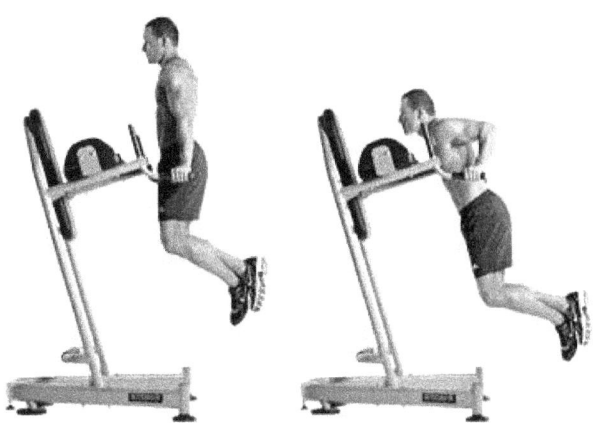

You will also find this one in the beginner's version of this workout. Make it more challenging by adding ankle weights to your ankles and pulling your knees up to your chest when you are in the up position.

Sample 12-Week Muscle Confusion Workout Plan

Here is a sample workout plan for 12 weeks that incorporates all the different workouts you need, the rest days you should be taking, and the periodic changes that you should be making.

It repeats after each 3 weeks (rather than the 4). Each week with a star (*) next to it is one in which you should change up at least 2 of the 5 variables that you read about earlier in this chapter.

This is a very general plan that you can adapt to your own needs and abilities.

It can be used with either beginner or intermediate workouts from steps 3, 4, and 5 of this book or your own preferred workouts.

The important thing is that you make sure to maintain this balance of resistance cardio (step 3), full body strength training (step 4), and muscle confusion workouts (step 5) in order to achieve maximum fat burning power.

Once you have worked through the full 12 weeks, you can start back at the beginning again and repeat the cycle.

Of course, by the end of those 12 weeks, you'll be in significantly better shape than you were when you started so you can up the intensity by adding more resistance, more weight, or longer high intensity intervals.

Adapt it to your skills as you progress so that you continue to see the amazing results that you want.

Others who are considering purchasing this book would love to know what you think. If you could spare a few seconds, they would greatly appreciate reading an honest review from you. Simply visit the page on Amazon.com.

	Sun	Mon	Tues	Wed	Thurs	Fri	Sat
1	Step 3	Step 3	Rest	Step 4	Step 5	Rest	Step 5
2	Step 4	Rest	Step 3	Step 4	Rest	Step 5	Step 5
3	Rest	Step 3	Step 3	Rest	Step 4	Step 4	Rest
4*	Step 3	Step 3	Rest	Step 4	Step 5	Rest	Step 5
5	Step 4	Rest	Step 3	Step 4	Rest	Step 5	Step 5
6	Rest	Step 3	Step 3	Rest	Step 4	Step 4	Rest
7*	Step 3	Step 3	Rest	Step 4	Step 5	Rest	Step 5
8	Step 4	Rest	Step 3	Step 4	Rest	Step 5	Step 5
9	Rest	Step 3	Step 3	Rest	Step 4	Step 4	Rest
10*	Step 3	Step 3	Rest	Step 4	Step 5	Rest	Step 5
11	Step 4	Rest	Step 3	Step 4	Rest	Step 5	Step 5
12	Rest	Step 3	Step 3	Rest	Step 4	Step 4	Rest

Step 6

STOP Making these 10 Mistakes Immediately

Working out - especially using the HIIT techniques you have been learning about - offers many benefits to your health and overall wellbeing. But it also can be risky if you don't do it properly.

There are a lot of myths and false information out there that lead many people to make mistakes during their workout.

Some of these mistakes keep you from getting the full benefit of your workout and others are just downright dangerous.

So make sure that you avoid falling into any of these 10 bad habits of working out:

Don't Lean on the Machine

Leaning on the treadmill, elliptical, or any other machine you are using for the cardio part of your workout will decrease the intensity of your workout which will, in turn, decrease the number of calories you burn.

It's ok to have a light grip on the handles to help you keep your balance when you need it but, as a rule, you should avoid holding on to the handles or console at all times so that your body weight remains on your legs.

If the intensity of your cardio workout is so much that you feel you can't get through it without leaning on the machine, knock it down a notch instead of leaning to get through it.

If you have to lean, it means you are taking on more than your body can handle. Avoid injury and help your body build up muscle more efficiently by lowering the intensity so your body can catch up.

Don't Forget to Add Resistance

A lot of people mistakenly think that increasing the incline on a treadmill or adding resistance on a stationary bike will make them bulk up more than they want to.

In fact, adding resistance is what helps you increase the number of calories you burn and increase your endurance. Increasing the incline on the treadmill is especially important because the treadmill is already propelling you forward so that you don't have to work as hard to keep running.

Increasing the incline will give you the workout intensity you need to burn the maximum number of calories.

Don't Stretch After the Warm Up

Stretching and warming up are not the same thing. Both are important but they do different things. Stretching should either be done before the warm up or after the whole work out (or before and after).

The warm up should be done right before the main warm up. The purpose of the warm up is to get your blood pumping, warm up your muscles and increase the amount of fluid in your joints.

Doing this lowers your risk of damaging your joints and muscles during the workout. If you go into stretching after your workout, you'll lose all the benefits of the warm up.

Don't Carry Weights during Your Walk

A lot of people will try to boost the intensity of their cardio routine by carrying weights while they walk. However, the amount of weight you would need to carry to make a real difference is far more than the 3-pound maximum recommended by the American Council on Exercise.

So boost the intensity by increasing the incline or resistance of your cardio routine rather than trying to carry weights. Alternate between strength training and cardio workouts if you're trying to get an even tone across the full body.

Don't Skimp on the Strength Training

Many people think of burning fat and building muscles as two mutually exclusive things. And in most cases, they think that cardio is the way to burn fat while strength training is the way to build muscle.

But the fact is, our bodies do not work like this. If you only do cardio because you are only trying to burn fat, you are quickly going to hit a workout plateau where your body gets stuck at a certain weight.

You need to have a balanced routine of cardio and strength training in order to get the full range of benefits that exercise has to offer.

The more muscle you have, the faster your body burns calories. This means strength training will give your body the extra push it needs to break past the plateau and continue burning those last few extra pounds.

Don't Dehydrate Yourself

Not only is dehydration a severe risk to your health; it can also make your workout less effective. Your muscles have to strain harder to accomplish the same intensity of workout if you do not have enough water.

The average person can lose as much as 32 oz. in sweat during a moderate to intense 60-minute workout. This means you need to make sure to drink plenty of water before and after your workout to make sure that loss doesn't lead to dehydration.

If your workout lasts longer than 60 minutes, you'll need to keep water with you and take 4-8 oz. drinks every 15-20 minutes. After your workout, you need to drink at least 16oz of water per pound lost.

That means you should weigh yourself before and after the workout to see how much you need to rehydrate yourself (preferably using the same scale).

Don't Do the Same Workout Every Day

One of the most common mistakes is doing the same thing over and over. We find a workout we like and just do it again and again until it becomes old hat.

Of course, you do need to find a workout that you enjoy so that you are more likely to stick with your workout plan. But that doesn't mean you should be doing the same thing day in and day out. Mix up your workout by adding a couple different routines to your weekly plan.

This will prevent you from getting bored, overtraining and injuring certain muscle groups (while neglecting others) and hitting a weight plateau before you reach your goal weight.

Don't Lose Focus

Some people watch TV or read while working out in order to help distract themselves from the intensity of the exercise or from the monotony of routine.

But distracting yourself means you are not focused on your workout, which means you are at a higher risk of slacking off and losing form.

You need to give your full attention to your body during your workout so that it stays in ideal form and you push yourself to your maximum effort.

This will boost the number of calories burned and increase all the other benefits as well. If you find yourself getting bored, do something new.

You can listen to music to keep yourself motivated but it's best to avoid anything that requires more mental capacity than that (like audio books or TV shows where you have to follow a plotline).

Don't Speed Up Your Weight Lifting Routine

Lifting weights too fast is extremely dangerous. From sprains to tears to overstraining; there are just too many things that could go wrong when you are lifting weights too quickly.

You need to go at a steady rate so that you can pay attention to form. If you want to blend a little cardio into your weight lifting routine, throw in some full body moves rather than increasing the speed.

Try some of the full body workout techniques mentioned in Step 4 or come up with your own variations to spice up your weight lifting routine.

Don't Count Every Activity as an Exercise

It is true that every activity you do (from loading the dishwasher to walking around the grocery store) will burn more calories than you would if you did not do that activity.

But that doesn't mean you can count it as exercise. It is important to be active throughout the day but you won't get the full range of benefits that you get from your workout just by being more active.

To count as actual exercise, it needs to elevate your heart rate for at least 10-20 consecutive minutes. To count as an elevated heart rate, it should be somewhere between 55% and 85% higher than your resting heart rate.

Step 7

Jump Start Your Metabolism with these 10 Tricks

Exercising, especially by using the HIIT method, is by far the best way to boost your metabolism to its maximum efficiency.

It also helps increase what your metabolism's maximum efficiency is. You have already read about many of the ways that your new workout routine will help to boost your metabolism and increase the number of calories you burn.

But there's still more that you could be doing to jump-start your metabolism and give it that added boost to really maximize the number of calories you are burning each day.

Here are 10 other habits you should practice each day in addition to your workout:

Drink Black Coffee

Coffee has gotten a bad rap in the past and it's definitely true that too much of it is bad for you. But recent studies are starting to show that 1-2 cups per day is not only safe, it is actually beneficial.

A cup of coffee will keep your metabolism elevated for 3 hours after you drink it. Drinking coffee with your meal will help you metabolize the meal faster than if you hadn't had coffee.

But remember - you don't need to (and shouldn't) drink gallons of coffee. In too high of a dose, caffeine can cause heart problems and increased blood pressure.

So keep it to 1 or 2 cups per day and never drink caffeinated beverages of any kind after 5pm. Having caffeine too late in the day will mess up your sleep schedule.

So have a small or regular sized mug with breakfast and maybe another one with your lunch and then stick to water, decaffeinated teas, and juices with no sugar added for the rest of the day.

If you aren't a fan of coffee's natural flavor, just skip it all together because if you drown your coffee in milk and sugar, you'll end up doing more harm than good.

The milk and sugar will lead to a sharp jump in your glucose levels which will cause that quick perk followed by a sharp crash in the early afternoon. One of the keys to burning calories efficiently is making sure your glucose levels stay more or less stable throughout the day.

Drink Water

Water is absolutely essential for burning calories (and for surviving in general). One tall glass of water (about 17 oz.) will provide an immediate 30% increase in your metabolic rate for about 30-40 minutes after drinking it.

So, drinking a 17oz glass of water every hour or so will keep your metabolism at a consistently higher level. Drinking one or two glasses before a meal can help curb your appetite and prevent you from binging.

All in all, if you drink about 2 liters of water each day, you can burn at least 400 additional calories. That's about the same as a 30-minute run!

Drink Green Tea

Green tea is widely known to be a great healthy alternative to that third cup of coffee or soda. It contains antioxidants and flavonoids, which are great for preventing heart disease, cancer, and stroke.

But green tea does more than just prevent illness (as if that alone wasn't enough to start drinking it); it also burns calories. One cup of green tea will help you burn an additional 60 to 100 calories.

It may not sound like much at first but it adds up quickly.

Considering one cup has no more than 2 calories, that's well worth the metabolic boost. Combined with these other metabolism boosting tricks, you can watch the calories disappear.

Cut Out Sugar

Simple sugars (like white refined sugar or that found in processed foods) are the number one culprit for weight gain. Eating sugar will lead to more fat gain than eating fat.

This is because simple carbohydrates are too easily absorbed by the body, meaning that you don't burn as many calories in digestion and you get one quick jolt to your blood glucose rather than a steady stream of glucose throughout the day.

When your glucose levels are high, your metabolism slows down.

The problem is that most of the sugars we eat come from foods that we don't think of as sweet.

Fast food burgers contain an unholy amount of sugar. So do most of the low fat or diet foods. To replace the loss of flavor from taking out the fat, most products just dump in sugar.

So skip the diet versions and stick with full fat versions of food. As you will see below, your body spends more calories burning fat than it does burning sugar (meaning that a diet with plenty of healthy fats could actually lead to more fat loss).

Load Up on Fiber and Unsaturated Fats

Fiber and unsaturated fats are great for your body for a lot of reasons.

Let's start with fiber:

Studies have shown that eating 35 to 45 grams of fiber per day will not only curb your appetite and keep you feeling fuller for longer; it will also lead to more and faster weight loss than a low fiber diet.

But that doesn't mean you should start swallowing fiber supplements.

Get your 35 to 45 grams by breaking it up across each of your meals throughout the day.

Another important note - if you currently eat a low fiber diet, gradually increase the amount of fiber over the course of 1-2 weeks to avoid excess gas or that bloated feeling.

You can do this by switching to whole fruits instead of juice; making veggies your main course and meat a side dish; switching all your grains to whole grains; or adding nuts and seeds to your diet as healthy, filling snacks.

Now for unsaturated fats:

You might think that it sounds counterintuitive to eat fat if you are trying to lose fat but certain fats are actually healthy and boost the number of calories burned.

Unsaturated fats (which include monounsaturated and polyunsaturated) lower bad cholesterol, clean out plaque from your heart, and keep your blood pumping.

All of this will contribute to a more effective workout and overall healthier body. Foods high in unsaturated fats include nuts, olive oil, coconut oil, avocados, and other delicious snacks.

Many of these foods also tend to be higher in protein and fiber, which contribute to feeling more satisfied after a meal, which will decrease the overall number of calories you eat in the first place.

Heat Things Up

If you have a taste for spicy foods, you are in luck because capsaicin (the compound that give hot peppers their spicy kick) has been proven to help people lose weight.

It works in two ways. First of all, a spicy meal will raise your metabolism 8% more than its non-spicy counterpart. Second of all, a spicy meal will keep you feeling full for a longer period of time so that you end up eating fewer calories in a day.

One study showed that people who ate an appetizer covered in hot sauce ate an average of 200 fewer calories at their next meal than those who didn't.

Combine the fewer calories with the 8% increase in metabolic rate and you're looking at a nice boost to your average number of calories burned!

So if you're not a fan of fiery dishes, it may be worth the effort to gradually adapt to them.

Eat More Protein

Protein rich diets are absolutely essential to both burning fat and gaining muscle. Protein rich meals keep you feeling fuller for longer than low protein meals.

The more calories you get from protein rich sources, the less total calories you will eat. Studies have shown that people who got at least 30% of their calories from protein ate about 450 calories less per day than those who ate less protein.

This led to an average loss of 11 pounds over 12 weeks (and that was without using any other dietary tricks or exercises!)

Beyond that, proteins are complex nutrients that require a lot of energy to fully digest and use. This means your body burns more calories just trying to metabolize protein than it would on other foods.

It also increases the number of calories burned by adding to your muscle. Protein is essential to building muscle and muscle burns a lot more calories than fat (even when you're not doing anything).

So building up your muscle with a high-protein diet and strength training will lead to more calorie burn than simply focusing on burning fat.

To get the maximum benefit from a protein rich diet, eat healthy proteins. Fish, poultry, beans, nuts, and whole grains are rich in protein without adding too many bad fats.

Don't Crash Diet or Starve Your Body

While the most fundamental rule of losing weight is burning more calories than you consume, you shouldn't focus your entire weight loss plan on eating less calories. Instead, focus on eating nutrient-rich calories and burning more of them through regular exercise.

Crash diets shock your body and throw your metabolism out of whack. If you keep switching from starvation to binge eating, your body is going to think you are in the middle of a famine which means that the food you do eat will immediately get stored as fat (to be saved for the next famine).

Starving your body of the healthy nutrients it needs (like protein or healthy fats) will keep you feeling weak, unsatisfied, and hungry throughout the day.

It's far better to eat a nutrient rich, balanced diet and focus on increasing exercise and cutting out empty calories (like junk foods, sodas, fast food, and all processed foods).

While your specific needs may vary depending on what your personal goals and health restrictions are, a widely recommended balanced diet is one where you get 30% of your calories from protein, 15-20% from unsaturated fats, and 50-55% from complex carbohydrates.

So rather than obsessively counting every calorie; focus instead on making changes to achieve that balance.

Get Plenty of Omega 3 Fatty Acids

Omega 3 fatty acids have been widely praised for a number of health benefits from a healthier heart to a healthier brain. But they also seem to help with weight loss.

A recent study on obesity showed that people who took omega 3 fish oil supplements daily and ran just 3 times per week (45 minutes each) lost an average of about 5 pounds after just 3 weeks.

These results came with absolutely no other changes to diet or lifestyle aside from the fish oil supplements and the 3 runs.

It is thought that the reason it works so well is that omega 3 fatty acids help increase the blood flow to the muscles (boosting the amount of energy burned in a workout) while also stimulating the enzymes in your blood that convert fat stores into energy.

This means that adding omega 3 fatty acids to your daily diet (either as food or in fish oil supplements) could lead to more than 5 extra pounds of fat loss per month!

Making all of these changes at once could be a major shock to your body and your daily routine so instead, try to do them one at a time.

Do a 10-week challenge and add a new trick each week until all 10 have become a regular part of your routine.

I hope you have learned something from this book so far and would greatly appreciate it if you could leave an honest review on Amazon.com.

Discover Scientifically-Proven "Shortcuts" & "Hacks" to Lose Weight FASTER (With Very Little Effort)

For this month only, you can get Linda's best-selling & most popular book absolutely free – *Weight Loss Secrets You NEED to Know.*

Get Your FREE Copy Here:
TopFitnessAdvice.com/Bonus

Discover scientifically-proven tips to help you lose weight faster and easier than ever before. With this book, readers were able to improve their weight loss results and fitness levels. So, it's highly recommended that you get this book, especially while it's free!

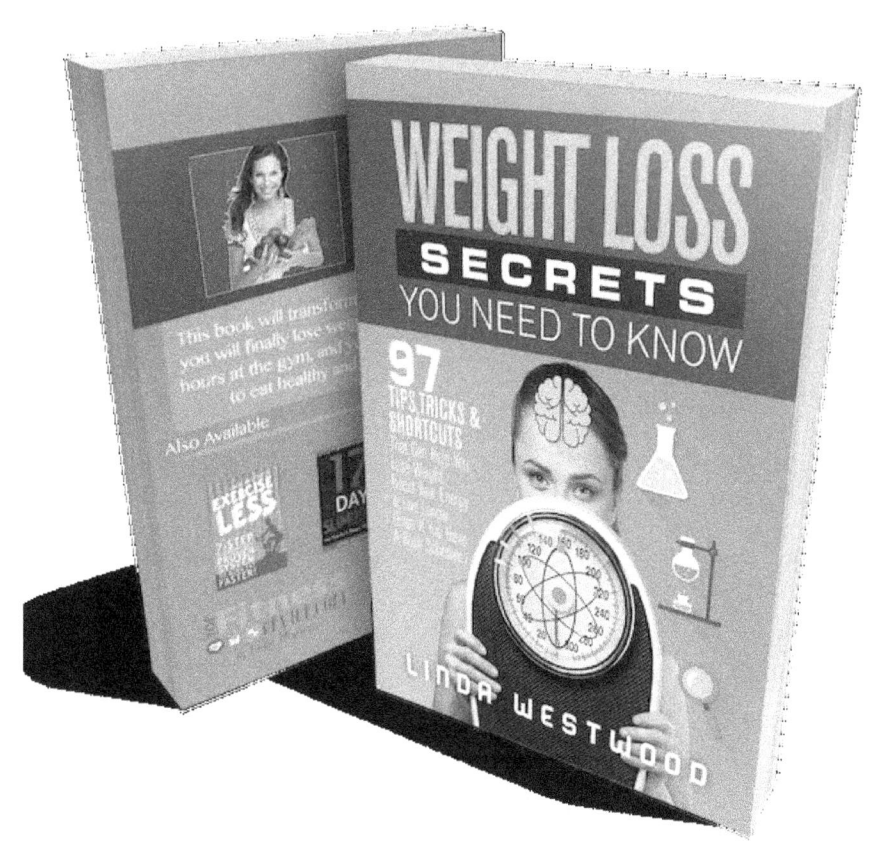

Get Your FREE Copy Here:
TopFitnessAdvice.com/Bonus

Conclusion

You might be sitting there right now thinking that making all of these changes is going to be an impossible feat. But that's the beauty of HIIT.

It is structured so that you do challenge yourself but you set those challenges at intervals so that you can accomplish them. As you progress, set the bar higher and higher.

As you master each of the 7 steps, the next step will be easier to take—not because the steps get easier but because *you* get stronger and more motivated.

By combining workouts from 3, 4, and 5 into your weekly routine, you'll be able to achieve total body transformation in a matter of weeks.

After the first week, you'll already notice yourself feeling stronger, lighter, and more energized. Plus, by maintaining variety with different workouts, you'll not only speed up muscle growth (and fat loss), you'll prevent yourself from getting bored.

Add the tips and tricks from steps 6 and 7 to add a further boost to your metabolism and prevent yourself from getting injured or unknowingly slowing your progress.

By the time you have achieved all 7 steps and made them part of your daily routine, you'll already feel like in your better shape than you have ever been in your entire life.

By the time you've incorporated each of the 7 steps into your new lifestyle, you'll have a newfound sense of strength, beauty, and accomplishment that you never knew possible and you'll find yourself wondering why you didn't start doing this years ago!

So now that you've finished reading, put this book down, get off that couch and take your first step toward the newer, stronger, more beautiful you!

Final Words

I would like to thank you for purchasing my book and I hope I have been able to help you and educate you on something new.

If you have enjoyed this book and would like to share your positive thoughts, could you please take 30 seconds of your time to go back and give me a review on my Amazon book page.

I greatly appreciate seeing these reviews because it helps me share my hard work.

You can leave me a review on Amazon.com.

Again, thank you and I wish you all the best!

Enjoying this book?

Check out my other best sellers!

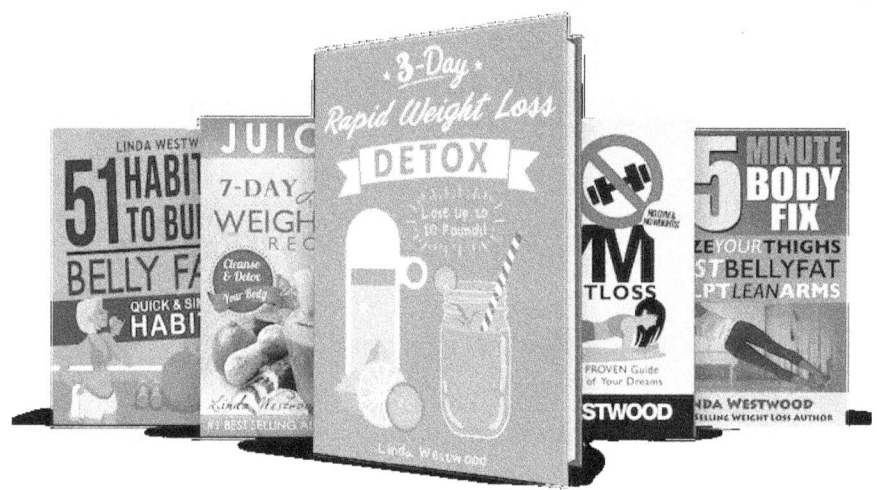

Get your next book on sale here:

TopFitnessAdvice.com/go/books

www.ingramcontent.com/pod-product-compliance
Lightning Source LLC
Chambersburg PA
CBHW031155020426
42333CB00013B/674